RUNNER'S WORLD™

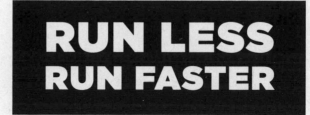

RUN LESS
RUN FASTER

RUNNER'S WORLD™

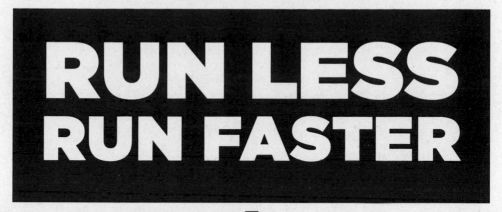

RUN LESS RUN FASTER

Become a Faster, Stronger Runner
with the Revolutionary
3-Runs-a-Week Training Program

Bill Pierce and Scott Murr

RODALE.

NEW YORK

Contents

In 2012, when I traveled to Greenville, South Carolina, to serve as a consultant to assist Furman University in its search for a head cross-country and track and field coach, I soon realized it was an ideal place for establishing a successful program. With its beautiful campus, local running trails, climate suitable for year-round training, outstanding academic reputation, and an administration eager for success, the university had it all. When the search committee asked if I would be interested, the opportunity to be in this ideal environment was enough to pull me from my head coaching position at my alma mater. No small factor in my decision was the opportunity to collaborate with the Furman Institute of Running & Scientific Training (FIRST).

Over the seven years that I have been at Furman University, FIRST has provided valuable metabolic and biomechanical assessments of our varsity runners as well as our professional running club, Furman Elite. As physiologists and runners, Bill Pierce and Scott Murr are enthusiastic supporters of our programs and their personal interactions with the athletes are greatly appreciated. Many of the runners have developed a strong interest in and knowledge of exercise science as a result of those interactions.

The tenets of the FIRST program coincide with our varsity coaching staff's training philosophy. FIRST places a strong emphasis on training at a pace that provides the runner with the stimulus to get better—the pace that brings about physiological adaptation. It is designing and implementing the FIRST program's paces that allows runners to remain healthy. That's exactly the same approach we take with our varsity athletes.

The FIRST program emphasizes the importance of strength training and flexibility. We spend about a third of our varsity practice time getting our runners stronger and more flexible. Cultivating this well-rounded athleticism is at the foundation of remaining healthy and being able to train consistently.

It's easy to see why runners following the FIRST Training Programs achieve personal records, and why so many are able to reach their goal of qualifying for the Boston Marathon. The FIRST philosophy of training with purpose includes the same basic principles that we incorporate with our varsity runners and the professional runners I coach.

It's a great pleasure working with Bill and Scott. I appreciate their many contributions to our Furman University cross-country and track programs. I strongly endorse their FIRST programs.

Now in its third edition, their best-selling book *Run Less Run Faster* is a valuable training tool for every runner.

Robert Gary
Two-time Olympian (Atlanta, 1996, and Athens, 2004)
Head Coach, Furman University Cross-Country and Track and Field Coach
Head Coach, USA Track and Field Men's Team at the World Championships, Doha, 2019

In 2005, Amby Burfoot, executive editor of *Runner's World* magazine, came to Greenville, South Carolina, to conduct interviews for an article he was writing about the Furman Institute of Running & Scientific Training (FIRST). During his visit, I showed him a collection of material that I planned to use to produce a training manual. As he perused the compiled resources, he insisted that the contents deserved a book, not just the spiral-bound manual I was proposing. A few months later, a New York City literary agent agreed with his assessment and in 2007, the first edition of *Run Less Run Faster* was published.

Because of its popularity, the first edition gave us many opportunities to speak at race expos, clinics, and professional meetings. At those engagements we met many midpack runners, as well as noted authors and elite runners. These interactions enabled us to learn more about what runners seek and how we might better meet their needs. When it came time to revise the original publication, we relied on the large compilation of frequent messages and valuable feedback we had received from runners on six continents over the years. The 2012 revised edition provided more details about how to use the FIRST Training Programs effectively.

Now we have received more than 10,000 messages relaying runners' successes, failures, and the unique challenges they may be facing. These requests reflect the need for specific situational advice and a sustained interest in the FIRST Training Programs. Once again, we felt compelled to update the book so that we could incorporate everything we've learned from runners since 2012—information gathered from the annual running clinics we conduct, the numerous presentations we make, and the thousands of messages we've received. In addition, we were eager to update the training programs for the Boston Marathon to be in accordance with the new qualifying times.

The guiding approach for the third edition is to provide as much of this specific how-to-train and race advice as possible. We used those personal scenarios that runners from all over the world have presented us with to craft specific advice in each chapter. Our goal is to eliminate the guesswork and indecision about what to do after pulling on your running shoes. It may be a third edition, but to us it's an extension of the training manual that we intended to create 15 years ago. We have added even more specific guidance about how to use the highly structured training programs with their detailed running workouts. We know from our coaching experience that runners like to be told exactly what to do and when to do it—and we also know that, left to their own devices, runners tend to neglect many other aspects of training that are vital to becoming a healthy, fast runner. This edition emphasizes how important it is to have a comprehensive training program for elevating fitness, getting faster, and increasing the likelihood of enjoying a long running career.

My coauthor, Scott Murr, and I have thoroughly enjoyed getting to know runners, hearing their stories, and learning from their experiences. Our correspondences, some stretching over many years, have also been enjoyable and informative. We have shared some of those messages in this book under the heading "Real Runner Reports," as we did in previous editions. Many readers have told us that they are inspired by these reports from other serious recreational runners.

Scott and I, along with our longtime running partner, Don Pierce, developed ideas for the three editions of this book over thousands of miles run together. Don has been involved in every aspect of the books we have written; not a table or word was cast without his feedback and scrutiny. As I did in the first two editions, I will serve as the voice of the book.

Bill Pierce

RUNNER'S WORLD™

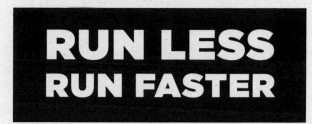

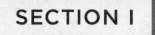

TRAINING
WITH PURPOSE

The FIRST 3Plus2 Training Program

Our running and coaching experiences prior to 2003 led us to the conclusion that many runners had goals, but that they did not have a defined pathway for achieving them. We regularly encountered runners who were frustrated in their futile attempts to get faster without any specific practical plan. Often, they assumed that they just needed to run more. Our motivation for founding the Furman Institute of Running & Scientific Training (FIRST) was to design a plan that non-elite runners could use to become healthier, to improve their running performance, to meet their challenging (but realistic) goals, and to avoid injuries. Further, we realized that most runners had a limited amount of time to train, so the training program had to fit into their way-too-busy lives.

Many runners have shared with us how the FIRST program came to their aid as they tried to find a path to meeting their goals and reaching their potential. No message captures that fulfillment and success better than the following email, received from Jo Linnane.

While I was sitting in my office in NYC, where I was an art director for a television show, a friend walked in and told me that she was running a 5K. I had been practicing karate for 20 years, but I was not a runner. The 5K promised a T-shirt and a beer at the end; I was in. I downloaded the "Couch to 5K" app. It took no time for the running bug to bite.

Soon I entered the NYC Marathon lottery and received one of the coveted spots. My goal, like that of many first-time marathoners, was to finish. With that goal accomplished, my dream running goal quickly changed. How could I get fast enough to qualify for Boston?

As a set designer and art director, I did not have a normal 9 to 5 schedule. I worked full time on a TV show and regularly designed 4 or 5 regional theater shows a year to satisfy my love of theater. That meant a lot of travel on top of a busy workweek. How could I fit marathon training into my busy professional endeavors?

After several marathons and lots of shorter races, I was getting faster. I targeted the Chicago Marathon for a Boston qualification. I trained very hard, using a five-days-a-week running plan. I approached the race with confidence, but crossed the finish line 6 minutes and 50 seconds short of qualification.

I pondered what I should do to reach my goal. I knew many people who ran even more miles than I did in a week. Should I? However, my body felt like it was in a perpetual bonk from training. I was either tired or injured. How could I tolerate even more?

A Facebook posting about my training and failed Boston attempt led another runner to tell me about a three-days-a-week training plan called FIRST. I wondered if actually running less might be the answer for me. It would fit with my busy professional life and maybe reduce my overall level of fatigue.

I decided to try the FIRST marathon training plan. I enjoyed the variety of the three demanding run workouts, and the recovery days provided relief from feeling perpetually pooped. Also, I avoided any serious running injuries while getting faster. I decided that the plan was a smarter way for me to train. The training fit well with my travel. I eas-ily fit the cross-training part of the FIRST training plan into my daily routine by heading to the gym before work or on the rare early day riding my bike in.

During the marathon preparation, I became more attuned to how my body responds to training. The test for the new approach to training came in Indianapolis. I was ecstatic when I crossed the line with a 10-minute PR and a Boston qualification.

Thank you, Bill and Scott.

Jo W. Linnane
Ogden, Utah

The core principles of the FIRST 3Plus2 Training Program value quality over quantity, with individualized training goals for every run. Because many runners are not able—physically or logistically—to run more than three times per week, the FIRST Training Program, based on three quality runs per week, have many adopters and endorsers around the globe.

We have received thousands of messages from runners who followed the FIRST Training Program for 16 weeks exactly as it was intended with remarkable results. They comment that they are now "believers," even though they were skeptical when they adopted the program. Usually, they add that their running friends told them that they would never improve while running less.

Our programs provide structure and specific paces tailored to each runner's current fitness level. The program, described later in this chapter, is grounded in a sound philosophy and scientific principles. Is it for everyone? We don't think that any single training program is for everyone. Each individual responds differently to training programs. History tells us that even elite runners have achieved their greatness with vastly different training methods. Is the FIRST Training Program the optimal way to train? We have never made that claim. What we have said is that it is an effective training program that works for many runners. The evidence of the program's success was solidly proven by studies that collected and examined physiological data, but also, and perhaps more importantly, by the thousands of Boston qualifications and other racing successes that runners who follow the program have earned.

Runners ranging from 2:40 to 6-hour marathoners tell us that the FIRST Training Program was central to their achievements. Many of the runners who say that they found success with the FIRST program had been injured in the past by following programs that required running daily or almost daily, or focused on high mileage. The FIRST program provided them with a means to participate injury-free in the sport that they had come to believe they could no longer enjoy. A large number reported to us that they have busy professional lives that do not permit them to run more often than the three Key Run workouts (an essential part of the FIRST Training Program) and, furthermore, that they were able to achieve their goals—typically, a Boston qualification—following the FIRST Marathon Training Program. Numerous clubs around the country have written us to say that their club uses this program because the specific structure of the workouts makes it easy to provide each club member with an individualized goal for each workout. We have learned that runners are disciplined and dedicated; they like structure and accountability. The FIRST Training Programs are designed to give you a specific distance and pace for each workout, based on your current level of running fitness.

The FIRST Training Programs are designed to produce optimal results with limited running. We have compressed our collective knowledge, experience, and research into a training method that provides specific workouts, laid out in 12- and 16-week training schedules for races from 5Ks to marathons (see Tables 6.1–6.5 in Chapter 6). These efficient and effective training programs have been tested with runners of wide-ranging abilities. Along with the training schedules, we include answers to many of the most frequently asked questions that we have received from runners around the world.

This book is based on the FIRST training philosophy of Training with Purpose. The chapters provide the essentials for becoming fitter and faster. We realize that it is unlikely that anyone has time to devote to an extensive regimen of strength training, flexibility, and cross-training. That's why we developed "The 7-Hour Workout Week," shown in Chapter 16, "Putting It All Together with the 7-Hour Workout Week." We offer a practical, detailed, and comprehensive training program that will keep you strong, flexible, and fit while not requiring much time. This basic program will enhance your running and contribute to keeping you a healthy, injury-free runner.

Likewise, we know that lengthy chapters on the complex topics of nutrition, environmental factors, and injuries can be more daunting than helpful. We offer simple nutritional guidelines and believe that you can become a healthy eater and a well-fueled runner by following our advice. Similarly, the information we share about training and environmental challenges is essential for coping with altitude, heat, cold, pollution, and other factors. Most importantly, we wish to help you stay healthy. All of our workouts and exercises are designed to help you avoid injury, while recognizing that running is a physical activity that requires repetitive movements of impact that contribute to overuse.

What Is the FIRST Philosophy?

At the heart of the FIRST philosophy is the belief that most runners do not train with purpose. When runners are asked to share their typical training week and the objective of each run, many are at a loss to explain why they do what they do. Not having a training plan that incorporates different distances, paces, and recoveries means that runners don't reach their potential. Nor do they garner maximum benefits from their investment in training time. The FIRST program makes the run workouts clear and specific, limits overtraining and burnout, and substantially cuts the risk of injury, while producing faster race times. By focusing on efficient, purposeful training, FIRST enables runners to meet their goal of running faster without sacrificing their job, family, friends, or health.

The FIRST 3Plus2 Training Program and Its Components

Three quality runs each week, plus two cross-training workouts, are the foundation of the breakthrough FIRST approach. Functional strength training and stretching are also essential parts of FIRST Training Programs. The three runs—the track repeats, the tempo run, and the long run—are designed to work together to improve endurance, lactate threshold, running pace, and leg speed. For each run, FIRST prescribes specific paces and distances that are based on the runner's current level of running fitness. The three quality runs, including prescribed paces and distances, are described in detail in Chapter 6.

Echoing our philosophy of Training with Purpose, having a specific goal for each training run is another of the program's innovations. If you don't know what you're training toward, how can you possibly get there?

FIRST's prescribed paces are usually reported by runners as being faster than their normal running speed. Generally, this is because our Training with Purpose philosophy favors quality over quantity, intensity over frequency, fast running over the accumulation of miles. If you want to race faster, you need to train faster. In addition to running less, what sets the FIRST program apart from other training programs is that it emphasizes a faster pace for the long runs than what other training programs typically recommend. In our studies, we've discovered that focusing on a designated, demanding pace for the long runs prepares runners physiologically and mentally for racing, particularly for the marathon. Studies in various sports show that competitive practices produce more focused competitors in games and competitions. The focus necessary to complete each FIRST Key Run workout makes runners stronger mentally in races.

The physiological value of this faster running is that it increases the muscles' ability to metabolize lactate. Why is this important? An accumulation of too much lactate inhibits the aerobic energy available for muscular action. By training at a higher intensity, the muscle adapts to the increased energy demand by developing the ability to use lactate as an energy source, rather than having it accumulate in the muscles and blood.

The FIRST Training Program also builds in more recovery time between running workouts than typical running programs do. Without sufficient recovery, it is difficult to complete quality run workouts. Muscles need time to recover from the stress of hard workouts. Stressing specific muscle fibers repeatedly, day after day, in the same pattern causes accumulated fatigue. In other words, running six miles five days a week results in muscular fatigue, not muscular adaptation. However, using those same muscle fibers for a different type of activity will permit recovery and recharging of the muscle's energy stores (glycogen). You can engage in another aerobic activity and reap the cardiorespiratory benefits while the muscle fibers used in running are recharging for the next hard running workout. Chapter 8 explains further the importance of rest and recovery.

Most other running programs ignore the benefits of cross-training in favor of running more miles. FIRST's cross-training workouts not only enhance fitness but also add variety, which ultimately reduces vulnerability to overuse injuries. Plus, your training will be more interesting. Cross-training workouts at prescribed intensities increase blood flow around muscles, which in turn increases the muscle's ability to utilize oxygen and fat as energy sources for exercise. Using fat as an energy source spares the limited stores of carbohydrates (glycogen). Therefore, cross-training provides the same benefit as the additional running miles of other typical running programs. In Chapter 7, the cross-training workouts that are an essential part of the 3Plus2 Training Program are described in detail.

Functional strength-training exercises for runners and stretches for the development and maintenance of good range of motion are shown in Chapters 14 and 15. To avoid injury while becoming a fit and fast runner, strength and flexibility are necessary. In Chapter 16, "Putting It All Together with the 7-Hour Workout Week," we show how to incorporate exercises and stretches in as little as 10 to 20 minutes per day.

Where's the Proof?

In 2003, when we established the Running Institute, we were convinced from our own experiences that these three running workouts, coupled with vigorous cross-training, would help runners improve both their race times and their overall health. We were eager to conduct training studies with a variety of runners to test our 3Plus2 Training Programs. We had designed the training programs to help runners train effectively, efficiently, and to avoid overtraining and injury. But could we prove that they were, in fact, doing all these things?

Exercise science studies that test the effectiveness of training regimens are typically conducted in laboratories where potentially confounding variables can be controlled. We stewed over how to design our studies. Many research studies use male college freshmen as subjects because professors have easy access to them. We wanted to test our programs on "real" runners—fast, slow, male, female, young, old, novices, or race veterans—performing their training without direct supervision. Our goal was to test a program that would enable us to generalize the results to the typical runner. That required our giving up control. We also wanted to find out if our program worked under the conditions that runners using our program would face—finding an accessible running track, having a measured running course for tempo and long runs, and being able to maintain a specific pace for a workout.

For three consecutive years, we conducted studies with 25 participants each, male and female participants from all over the country, ranging in ages from 23 to 63, who agreed to follow the FIRST Training Program for 16 weeks. Each study began with the participants being tested in the laboratory to assess their fitness. After following the 16-week training program, they returned for repeat testing. In addition to the laboratory assessments, in the latter two studies, the participants also ran a marathon. In all three studies, the runners showed significant improvement over the 16 weeks of training. All three variables critical to running performance—maximal oxygen consumption, running speed at lactate threshold, and running speed at peak oxygen consumption—improved by following a three-quality-runs-per-week training program. We now had data to support our personal experiences. And, most important to the runners themselves, each improved on at least one of the running performance variables. A summary of the studies' results is reported later in this chapter.

The three-quality-runs-per-week training program enabled all the first-time marathoners to finish, very much satisfied with their performance times. More impressive were the personal best times recorded by more than 70 percent of the veteran marathoners. Running only three days a week, coupled with two cross-training workouts each week, enabled even veteran marathoners, who were accustomed to running five or six days a week, to improve their physiological profiles from the laboratory assessment, as well as improving their marathon performances.

Although the studies supplied strong proof that the training programs were effective and led us to write *Run Less Run Faster*, we believe that the evidence provided by the many successes reported over the past 15 years is even stronger proof that the FIRST training approach is effective. Having runners follow the program on their own, rather than having us monitor their workouts and provide them with feedback, is a strong endorsement that the program can be used by runners without direct coaching. Receiving reports from runners who describe how they followed the program, as laid out in the book, and subsequently ran a personal best time or achieved a Boston qualifying time indicates that the programs not only have the key elements needed to get fitter and faster, but that runners are able to self-coach with the training programs in the book. Further evidence for the effectiveness of the FIRST Training Programs is that those reporting success represent a wide range of abilities, ages, experience, both female and male, from six continents.

Training with Purpose means having workouts designed to specifically target the determinants of running performance. These studies and the countless success stories indicate that our 3Plus2 Training Programs are not an empty promise. Runners tend to have more confidence in methods that other runners have used successfully. The FIRST Training Programs also provide the structure and accountability that runners like by specifying both distance and pace for each workout, so there is a clear measure of performance for each training run. Running six miles is one thing; running six miles only 30 seconds slower than 10K pace is quite another.

Can All Runners Benefit from the FIRST Training Programs?

Our research studies say yes for age-group runners; however, we have not tested it with national and world-class runners. These training programs were designed for regular runners aspiring to improve their running. The FIRST Training Programs have been used to improve running performances by five-hour marathoners and sub–three-hour marathoners, by runners preparing for their first 5K or marathon, and by beginning runners in their early 20s as well as veterans in their 70s and 80s. In addition, the 3Plus2 Training Programs are extremely flexible and can be adjusted to fit the needs of all types of runners, from those who have limited time to train, to those who make training a major focus in their lives.

Results of the Three Studies

Pre- and post-training, three variables were compared to determine the effects of the 16-week training program: (1) VO_2 max (maximal oxygen intake), (2) running speed at lactate threshold, and (3) running speed at peak VO_2. The results are displayed in the summary table (Table 1.1). You can see that, as a group in all three studies, the runners showed improvement over the 16 weeks of training on all three variables related to running performance, all statistically significant. Individually, all runners improved on at least one of the running performance variables.

TABLE 1.1

Summary of Results from Three FIRST Studies

(Runners in the 2003 study did not run a marathon at the end of the study. They were assessed only in the lab.)

	2003	2004	2005
Females	7	10	8
Males	15	12	9
Ages (years)	23–63	25–56	24–52
Average Age (years)	F = 41.7 M = 40.1	F = 34.8 M = 36.7	F = 35.0 M = 35.4
% Improvement of VO$_2$ max	4.8	4.2	5.4
% Improvement of Running Speed at Lactate Threshold	4.4	2.3	5.6
% Improvement of Running Speed at Peak VO$_2$	7.9	2.4	2.1
Range of Marathon Finish Times for Females		3:56–4:44	3:41–4:49
Average Marathon Finish Times for Females		Median = 4:17:02 Mean = 4:20:42	Median = 3:56:18 Mean = 4:02:22

	2003	2004	2005
Range of Marathon Finish Times for Males		2:56–4:51	2:27–4:19
Average Marathon Finish Times for Males		Median = 3:46:19 Mean = 3:49:23	Median = 3:42:51 Mean = 3:35:24
Number of First-Time Marathon Finishers		8 (3F, 5M)	3 (2M, 1F)
Average Time of First-Time Marathoners		F(3) = 4:03:07 M(5) = 3:48:49	F(1) = 4:03:34 M(2) = 3:46:22
Number of Personal Best Times (for those who had run a marathon previously)		7 of 13 (53.8%)	12 of 14 (85.7%)

REAL RUNNER REPORT

Dear Bill and all at Furman,

I have emailed you over the years in praise of your marathon plans, so I hope that you will indulge me another, slightly longer email.

In 2014, at the age of 50, I ran 3:09 at the Nottingham Marathon, after following your *Run Less Run Faster* plan. I was delighted with this run, with a negative split and my best marathon time for 5 years (all my marathons have been via your plan). Some of my running companions said that with higher running mileage, I would be able to run under 3 hours, even at the age of 50. Unfortunately, I succumbed to their suggestions. I gradually began replacing my cycling workouts with running workouts to increase my running mileage over the winter of 2014–15. I developed terrible pain in my left hip. I continued training but, during a 10-mile run, the pain was so bad that I had to walk the final 4 miles. The next morning I could hardly get out of bed. I took a few days off and tried again, with the same result. And this became the pattern of my running until I could stand it no longer. I went to see my doctor, who diagnosed trochanteric bursitis. I was prescribed some strong NSAIDs, but stopped taking them after a few days as I did not like the side effects.

I decided to stop running altogether and took 4 months off and picked up with cycling again—a sport that I have done since my teens. In the summer of 2015, with no more hip pain, I started a run/walk programme to see if I could get back into running. I found that I could run 10–15 miles a week, but any more would cause pain in my left hip. Oh well, I thought, such is the state of the aging runner.

This is where your *Train Smart, Run Forever* comes in. I read a review of the book in *Runner's World* and ordered my own copy, which I read from cover to cover. Some of the runners' anecdotes matched my own experiences. So I started following your 7-hour workout week. I realised that what had been missing from my running was properly structured strength training. Gradually, I found that I was able to increase my running mileage and felt stronger and faster than I had done since my hip injury. I ran a hilly 10K in 42:04, took care to recover and had no pain. I decided to follow the 10K plan from your original *Run Less Run Faster*, replacing the KW1 with the Tuesday run from TSRF. I ran the Boxing Day 10K in 41:04, a full minute quicker in only 2 months. Again, I took care to recover properly. I decided to follow the full RLRF 10K plan, including the KW1 track repeats—but I kept to the structure of the 7-hour workout week.

Last week, I competed in the Northumberland Coastal Trail Race. This race is 6.5 miles along coastal trails and beaches, with plenty of hills. I have to tell you that, thanks to your plan, I won this race outright in 44:41. There were 200 competitors; and maybe the quality of the field was not up there; and I have always been strong over cross-country.

But I have to say thank you, thank you, thank you for your running plans. I had reached the stage of retiring from running altogether, but now, in my 55th year, I know that your plans will help me to keep running forever.

Jonathan Fish
Head Teacher
Lancaster, United Kingdom

2

Principles of Training

There are five primary principles of training that apply to runners. These five principles should be incorporated into any training program. FIRST Training Programs adhere to these five basic training principles.

Principle #1: Progressive Overload

The gradual increase of training stress causes the body to adapt in response to the overload. These adaptations occur at the cellular level and this adaptation process will continue as long as the overload does not overwhelm the body. That is why the additional stress—increased exercise time and intensity—must be added gradually. Adequate recovery time must be allowed before the next stress overload.

Principle #2: Specificity

The improvement from training is specific to the type of training. Specificity applies to the mode (type) of exercise, intensity (speed or pace), and duration (distance or total time run). That's why 5K and marathon training differ.

Obviously, to become a better runner you need to run. The question is how much of your training needs to be mode-specific. The FIRST program specifies a smaller percentage of your total training to be running than other running programs. As we explain throughout the book, our experience and research show that a high level of fitness and running success can be achieved by running three times a week.

The FIRST training approach adheres to the principle of specificity for intensity. We advocate that, to run faster, you must incorporate faster running into your training. Runners report that the FIRST training paces are challenging. Runners also report that running fast in training helps them run faster in races more than running more frequently in training. Pace-specific training is the primary basis of FIRST training.

Principle #3: Individual Differences

Runners will soon find that they progress at different rates from those of their training partners. Individuals are different in their anatomies and physiologies, and respond differently to the same training stimulus. It is important for you to focus on your own progress—where you are now, as opposed to where you were or where you will be three months from now. There will always be others who are fitter and faster, and others who are not as fit or as fast. The principle of individual differences also applies to rest and recovery. Some runners can bounce back from a high-quality track workout or an intense tempo run sooner than other runners.

Principle #4: Law of Diminishing Returns

One of the benefits of being a novice is that your early progress is substantial. As you progress through the training programs and you get fitter and faster, you are approaching your optimal performance. As you near that point, small improvements come from lots of hard training, as opposed to the large improvements that came from moderate training when you were first beginning.

Principle #5: Reversibility

Use it or lose it! The gains that you make can be lost if you stop training. Consistency is the key to fitness. It's easier to stay in shape than to get in shape.

FIRST encourages regular year-round training. That is one of the attractive features of running three times per week. The rigors of daily running may cause some runners to stop running for long periods, and interruptions in regular physical activity cause a loss of fitness that leads us to try to make up for those losses too fast once we return to training. But runners following the FIRST program are less likely to get overwhelmed or burned out from running. The training does not have to be at full intensity year-round; low to moderate intensity can help you maintain fitness and not be susceptible to the stress and injuries that come from sudden increases in physical activity.

||||||

REAL RUNNER REPORT

Dear Drs. Pierce and Murr,

I have to take a moment to thank you for your excellent book, *Run Less Run Faster*. I am by all means a recreational athlete, and my full-time job as a resident physician translates to a busy schedule with sometimes irregular and long hours.

I trained with the 3:35 plan, knowing that for my age group I'd have to be even a bit faster (I'm 31). I just ran the Portland Marathon on October 9 in a new PR by over 8 minutes, finishing in 3:30:10—my first BQ!! Prior to reading this book I was the epitome of a junk mileage runner—I ran four marathons last year (prior PR 3:38:53), and did a half-Ironman. My last race of the year was CIM in Sacramento and it ended horrendously. I was exhausted and was actually getting worse.

After taking some time off to enjoy other things like CrossFit, I got it in my head that if I dedicated myself to an actual training plan, I MIGHT be able to qualify for Boston. It felt unrealistic but I had to admit that a BQ was what I wanted more than anything. As a physician, I liked the evidence and science you presented, and your book resonated with me. After sticking to it (I won't lie, I hated my first track workout), I have almost a 5-minute cushion for the 2018 race!

My first marathon in 2009 was a 4:23, so this is a huge progression and has boosted my confidence tremendously. In fact, one week after the race, I signed up for my first Ironman in Boulder, June 11, 2017. Maybe it was just the post-race endorphins still circulating, but you helped me meet my number-one goal so I needed a new one. I look forward to following a similar plan as I train for my next triathlon.

Sincerely,

Stephanie Go, MD
Department of Radiology
Stanford University Hospitals and Clinics

AN UPDATE: _____

Since I first wrote to you three years ago, I've qualified for Boston 3 times—including this year with the new, faster requirements! (New PR of 3:27:01 this summer.)

Additionally, I've finished 3 full Ironmans and a bunch of other shorter triathlons since then. Thanks for the suggestions to start cross-training! Amazing what you can accomplish when you only run 3 days a week. I finally completed residency and fellowship as well, and am now practicing full time as a radiologist in Portland, OR.

Best of luck with the new edition! My current copy is dog-eared, highlighted, and annotated.

My sister and husband used it to run their first marathons, and my best friend is a convert too after too many injuries.

Thank you again!!!

3

Realistic Goals

Runners who attend FIRST Retreats and those who write to us want to know if their goals are realistic. They want us to tell them what race times they are capable of running now and what race times they can expect to run in the future. Based on their training times and, in the case of those who have visited our laboratory, their physiological profile, we can provide a fairly accurate estimate of what a runner is physiologically capable of running. However, we don't have a crystal ball and cannot provide a future prediction with certainty. That's what makes entering races so much fun.

There are numerous variables that determine race performances; not all of them can be nicely quantified by means of a metabolic analyzer. However, the more data we have to consider from lab and field tests, the better we can help the runner set realistic goals.

In particular, marathon time prediction is difficult. Expected times for shorter races, from 5Ks to half-marathons, are fairly predictable, assuming that the runner chooses a realistic pace and has prepared appropriately for the distance. Perhaps the allure of the marathon is related to its uncertainty. Don't you love watching a game that comes down to the final minute of play with the outcome undetermined? Uncertainty is the element of sport that contributes to its popularity. I believe that the same is true of the marathon.

I am seldom, if ever, surprised by the outcome of a 5K, 8K, 10K, 10-mile, or half-marathon race. I know within seconds what I will be able to run. With the marathon, it's a mystery. Even during the race, whether you are halfway, at 20 or 24 miles, you won't know what is going to happen during these final miles.

Many variables impact marathon performance. You battle physical challenges, such as maintaining core temperature and fuel stores, muscle fatigue, and orthopedic stress, all the way to the finish line. Any one of those factors can undermine great preparation and a good performance in a race. Changes in environmental conditions, such as temperature, headwinds, or humidity, also may spoil your best-laid plans.

Marathoners who fail to achieve their goal finish time immediately begin to question their preparation and training. In many cases, their preparation was good and appropriate, but the runners may have been unlucky because one of the many variables noted above was not optimal on that day. However, setting an unrealistic finish-time goal that is just a couple of minutes too ambitious, particularly in the marathon, will lead to a too fast early pace that will undermine good preparation and a great effort.

Why is it that runners are disappointed with race finish times? Often, it is not because of a poor performance, but it's the result of their having set unrealistic goals. For example, a runner who just finished a 10K in 40:30 might be despondent because she had hoped to run under 40:00. It very well may be that she just ran a superb race. That is, based on her 5K and half-marathon times, her predicted 10K time was 41:00, which means she ran five seconds per mile faster than what was predicted. She had a remarkable performance from what had to be a great effort, but her expectations simply prevented her from enjoying and appreciating it.

The question to ask is this: Why and how did she establish 40:00 as her target finish time for the 10K? Most likely, her disappointment is a result of wanting to be a "thirty-something" 10K runner, just as runners want to be a "three-something" or "two-something" marathoner. If I had been coaching her, I would have told her that, based on her recent performances at these other race distances and on her training paces, running 10 seconds per mile faster than what was predicted was unlikely and trying to do so would likely result in her fading over the last couple of miles. I would have said, "Let's set three goals for your 10K: (1) 41:15, acceptable run, representing a good effort; (2) under 41:00, faster than predicted, representing a very good performance; and (3) sub-40:45, outstanding effort and performance."

As it was, her better-than-predicted excellent time of 40:30 represented an outstanding effort, but she was disappointed because she had not set a realistic goal. She could have benefited from good coaching advice. That's why we have placed this important topic so early in this book.

Of course, we want to encourage runners to challenge themselves and set ambitious goals. However, running too fast early in the race because you chose an overly ambitious, unrealistic goal almost always leads to dire consequences in the second half of the race. You'll be disheartened when an outstanding performance is unsatisfying because you chose an arbitrary and unrealistic goal.

I find that many of the runners applying to FIRST for coaching have unrealistic goals. At least, they are unrealistic in the short term. They may be able to reach their goals with steady and wise training over a period of one to two years. Many expect miracles in 16 weeks. These unrealistic goal times occur when runners select them arbitrarily, usually round numbers or, in many cases, a qualifying time, such as that for the Boston Marathon. The ability of FIRST to help runners set realistic goals is just as valuable as our individually tailored training programs.

How do runners undermine their own performance? Consider this example. A runner with a 5K race finish time of 22:00 has a predicted marathon time of 3:34:05 (using Table 3.1). If the runner sets 3:30 as a goal, he will need to run nearly 10 seconds faster per mile than the pace necessary to run a 3:34:05. Attempting to run 10 seconds per mile faster for 26.2 miles than what your current fitness level indicates will most likely result in a disappointing finish, and you'll end up questioning what element was missing in your training program. But the only thing missing was a realistic goal.

Realistic Goals: Q & A

Q. *How does the selection of the goal finish time affect your performance?*

A. Selecting a goal finish time that's too ambitious will cause you to run too fast during the early miles of the race. That fast start will likely result in a slower pace in the latter part of the race and a disappointing finish time.

Q. *If my 10K time predicts a 3:13 marathon, is it OK to set 3:10 as my goal?*

A. Running three minutes faster than your predicted marathon finish time means running seven seconds faster per mile than the pace that is presumably representative of your current fitness level. For most marathoners, running seven seconds per mile faster for the entire distance would be challenging and most likely not realistic. Trying to do so could lead to a disappointing finish time.

Q. *Would it be reasonable to expect an improvement over a 16- to 18-week training period that would make the 3:10 in the previous question possible?*

A. Absolutely. That's why we train. While there are no guarantees, due to numerous variables (weather, course, personal health, etc.), a good marathon training program can produce that result. We have had runners in our training programs make much bigger improvements. For the purpose of setting a revised goal, don't assume that improvement has occurred without confirmation from a shorter race or improved training times. In particular, we rely on long run training times to judge a runner's improvement and her potential marathon performance; we use tempo training times to determine a runner's improvement and her potential 5K and 10K goal times. Your improvement will depend on the type of training that you have done in the past.

Q. *What distance is the best predictor? What if the 5K and 10K predict different marathon finish times?*

A. The distance closest to the planned race distance is going to be the better predictor, assuming that the races were run under similar conditions. That is, a 10K is a better predictor of your marathon finish time than a 5K race finish time, and a half-marathon finish time will be a better marathon predictor than the 10K time.

If your 5K predicts a faster marathon time than what you are able to run, it is an indicator that your running speed is currently better than your running endurance and you need to concentrate on your longer runs. Conversely, if your marathon finish time predicts a faster 5K time than you are able to run, you need to work on speed and leg turnover.

Q. *Are the prediction tables accurate for everyone?*

A. Individuals differ in their abilities. Some runners have more speed than endurance and vice versa. For some runners, their 5K finish times will predict a faster marathon than what they can run, while for others, their marathon times are faster than what their 5K times predict.

Q. *Are there differences in the tables for men and women?*

A. Generally, women will run faster for longer distances and men faster for shorter distances. That is, if you have a man and a woman with the same 5K time, the woman will likely run a faster marathon than the man. Conversely, if you have a man and a woman with the same marathon time, the man will likely run a faster 5K than the woman.

Q. *Does age make a difference in the prediction tables?*

A. Aging runners usually have more endurance than speed. If a 55-year-old runner and 20-year-old runner have the same 5K time, it is likely that the 55-year-old would run the faster half- or full marathon. Conversely, if the 55-year-old and the 20-year-old had the same marathon time, the 20-year-old would likely have a faster 5K time. Older and experienced runners tend to be more economical and younger runners have more speed. From reviewing race results and single-age world records, we have found that older women (55 and older) tend to slow at an accelerated rate as compared to men. Perhaps these race results and records will change as more women with a longer history of competing become older.

Q. *How does the course profile affect the goal finish time?*

A. The fastest road racing times in the world at all distances have been set on flat courses with few turns (Berlin, Rotterdam, Chicago). Hills, turns, and rough or uneven surfaces all tend to slow the pace. While many runners will say that a flat course is boring and that they welcome a change to the repetitive, concentrated muscular contractions, there is a time cost for those changes. There are no clear measures to determine the time cost of specific elevation changes. Rolling hills may make the course more interesting and fun to run, but they may not contribute to a faster finish time. Often, there are website forums where veteran runners of a race will estimate what the time difference is for a specific race course, as compared to that for a flat course. Those postings by past participants in the race usually provide more helpful and accurate descriptions of a race course and its difficulty than the race's website.

Q. *Does my predicted finish time from the tables assume that there will be some elevation changes in the race?*

A. Assume that the finish-time prediction is valid if the race that you are using to predict your finish time at another distance is similar in terrain to that race. That is, if you ran a hilly 5K and you are using that race time to predict your half-marathon time on a hilly course, it is likely to be a reasonable predictor. However, if you ran a perfectly flat 10K and are using that time to predict your finish time on a hilly marathon course, then you should add time to that prediction to compensate for the additional time required for running the hills, depending on the length and steepness.

Q. *How do environmental conditions influence goal finish time?*

A. Ideal racing temperatures for most runners range from 40°F to 60°F (5°C to 16°C). A general estimate is that for every degree above 60°F you will slow by one second per mile in the marathon. We have provided heat-adjusted training times in Chapter 9. Of course, there are wide individual variations, based on sweat rates and body size. Smaller runners, who are able to dissipate heat better than larger runners, have the advantage in the heat, but are disadvantaged in colder temperatures. The extra energy cost of maintaining body temperature depends on the length of the race and your body size. Even light winds on a cool day (less than 60°F, or 15°C) can increase demands on the body for maintaining normal body temperature. Needless to say, having a race day with the ideal temperature, humidity, and winds is a rare treat for the runner. Look what those once-in-a-century ideal conditions produced at the 2011 Boston Marathon. Compare those with the scorching heat at the 2012 Boston Marathon or the cold rain and 25 mph winds in 2018. Unpredictable environmental conditions are just one additional factor making the determination of realistic goals a challenge. Do not fool yourself by thinking that you will defy environmental conditions and their effects on physiology; you won't.

Q. *As I get older my race times are slower. Is there a way to determine comparable times at my present age to those that I ran when I was younger?*

A. Yes. World Masters Athletics (WMA) has developed tables that adjust performances for aging. The age-graded factors and standards were developed based on the world records for that single year age. By comparing your time for a specific distance with the world best performance by a runner of your age, you can calculate a performance percentage. This percentage can be used to compare your performance to other runners or even to your own race performances at a younger age. It is a method for aging runners to set realistic goals.

Aging and Goal Setting

As runners hit the "big 4-0," friends and family will send cards celebrating being "over the hill." In reality, however, most runners will joke about being older, but most do not experience any decline in their training and racing. In fact, I ran my marathon PR at 41, almost 42. However, somewhere in the fourth decade, runners will begin to see slight declines in race performances that necessitate a change in goal expectations. That's why runners need to understand how goal setting is influenced by aging.

While the FIRST Training Programs were designed and have been effective for runners of all ages, they have been particularly popular with older runners. As runners age, they need more recovery and that typically leads to reduced training volume. Much research is being conducted on older runners. Whether the research is focused on mental or physical functioning, the results are clear that the key to good health and performance is to stay active and to do so consistently, so as to stave off the deterioration that we once thought was inevitable. Let's be clear: Running performance will decline with aging, except perhaps for those who began running late in life. However, the performance reductions predicted in the literature are being defied by a generation of runners who have maintained their intense training for decades.

Aging runners rarely escape without injury. As connective tissue becomes less supple and more susceptible to injury, tendonitis from inflammation is a common occurrence. After an injury that might sideline the older runner for weeks or months, fitness is lost and the attempt to regain it too fast leads to another injury and a vicious cycle of injury and recovery develops. This can lead to a more serious injury or a loss of motivation, both of which can lead you to become a former runner. That status contributes to weight gain and accompanying medical conditions associated with being sedentary. It's important to find a way through treatment and rehabilitation of an injury to maintain your fitness.

As runners' times begin to slow, there may be a loss of motivation to train intensely. In a *New York Times*[1] article about aging, Dr. Hirofumi Tanaka, an exercise physiologist at the University of Texas, recommended training intensely to improve oxygen consumption. In the same *Times* article, Dr. Steven Hawkins, an exercise physiologist at the University of Southern California, said that when you have to choose between hard and often, choose hard; in other words, intensity over frequency is the recommendation. He added, "High performance is really determined more by intensity than volume. Sometimes when you're older, something has to give. You can't have both so you have to cut back on the volume. You need more rest days." These two exercise physiologists' advice echoes the philosophy central to the FIRST Training Programs.

Training consistently is the key for aging runners because it is much easier to maintain fitness than to get fit as you age. While the times on the watch may represent slower performances, it is the intensity of the effort that matters. Yes, performances will decline, but serious training will reduce these inevitable decrements by 50% or more.[2] Runners who continue to train seriously will typically experience racing decrements less than 1% per year from their late 30s to their mid-40s. The slower performance times will most likely occur sooner in the shorter races—5K to 10K—than in the longer races. Marathoners can still run their best times in their late 30s and early 40s. For runners who sustain their training, performance losses in the 0.5% to 1% range can be expected from the mid-40s to the mid-50s. The slowing of performance times accelerates after age 55 with annual performance decrements ranging from 1% to 2.5%.[3]

The aging literature about runners is being rewritten as the baby boomers march into old age. FIRST is pleased that its programs have enabled runners in their 60s, 70s, and 80s, whose old ways of training had led to slower times and a loss of motivation, to report a renewed excitement with their training, along with improved age-group times. Masters age-adjusted calculators can provide age-adjusted times so that older runners can determine their running times' equivalences to those run at a younger age and set realistic goals appropriate for their age.

The authors have promoted running as a healthy lifelong physical activity by conducting more than 25 educational running workshops, based on scientific principles. The workshops are designed for runners who wish to optimize their training, maximize their running performance, and minimize injuries. Hundreds of runners have traveled from 40 states and 12 countries to attend one of these annual running workshops.

It is common for the runners who attended these workshops to list "running into old age" as their primary goal. In addition to their desire for lifelong running, they also point out that weight management and race participation supply motivation for continuing to train. The running workshop is conducted to provide age-group runners with the information needed to maintain and improve their running performances and to enjoy lifelong running.

The four-day running workshop provides physiological and biomechanical assessments for each participant. Runners complete a maximal oxygen consumption (VO_2 max) and lactate threshold (LT) test, along with an assessment of body composition (BodPod or DXA) and running gait. In addition to the extensive laboratory assessment, participants attend lectures on nutrition, strength training, cross-training, stretching for flexibility, injury prevention, good running form, smart racing strategies, and designing an effective training plan. They also participate in activities with an instructor demonstrating proper form and technique. Each participant receives an individualized training plan following completion of the workshop. The comprehensive nature of the running workshops is the most common reason given for the participants' decisions to attend the workshops.

We surveyed the runners to see if they were achieving their goals of "running into old age." Even though most of these runners are now in their 60s and 70s, 90% of the past workshop attendees were still running. The runners who attend the workshops are not elite runners, but they are committed to remaining physically active. In most cases, the 10% who are no longer running experienced an injury that prevented them from continuing to run. Most of those no longer running continue to be physically active with aerobic cross-training and other modes of physical activity.[4]

We concur with the workshop participants that "running into old age" is a positive goal. Is it realistic? With smart, consistent training, along with a healthy lifestyle, we believe it is.

TABLE 3.1

Race Prediction Table (Equivalent Performances)

Use the table to determine comparable performance times for four popular racing distances. The comparability assumes that you are properly trained for that distance.

5K	10K	Half-Marathon	Marathon
16:00	33:29	1:14:10	2:35:42
16:10	33:49	1:14:56	2:37:19
16:20	34:10	1:15:42	2:38:57
16:30	34:31	1:16:29	2:40:34
16:40	34:52	1:17:15	2:42:11
16:50	35:13	1:18:01	2:43:48
17:00	35:34	1:18:48	2:45:26
17:10	35:55	1:19:34	2:47:03
17:20	36:16	1:20:20	2:48:40
17:30	36:37	1:21:07	2:50:18
17:40	36:58	1:21:53	2:51:55
17:50	37:19	1:22:40	2:53:32
18:00	37:40	1:23:26	2:55:10
18:10	38:01	1:24:12	2:56:47

5K	10K	Half-Marathon	Marathon
18:20	38:21	1:24:59	2:58:24
18:30	38:42	1:25:45	3:00:02
18:40	39:03	1:26:31	3:01:39
18:50	39:24	1:27:18	3:03:16
19:00	39:45	1:28:04	3:04:54
19:10	40:06	1:28:50	3:06:31
19:20	40:27	1:29:37	3:08:08
19:30	40:48	1:30:23	3:09:45
19:40	41:09	1:31:09	3:11:23
19:50	41:30	1:31:56	3:13:00
20:00	41:51	1:32:42	3:14:37
20:10	42:12	1:33:28	3:16:15
20:20	42:32	1:34:15	3:17:52
20:30	42:53	1:35:01	3:19:29
20:40	43:14	1:35:47	3:21:07
20:50	43:35	1:36:34	3:22:44
21:00	43:56	1:37:20	3:24:21
21:10	44:17	1:38:07	3:25:59
21:20	44:38	1:38:53	3:27:36
21:30	44:59	1:39:39	3:29:13
21:40	45:20	1:40:26	3:30:51
21:50	45:41	1:41:12	3:32:28
22:00	46:02	1:41:58	3:34:05
22:10	46:23	1:42:45	3:35:42
22:20	46:44	1:43:31	3:37:20
22:30	47:04	1:44:17	3:38:57
22:40	47:25	1:45:04	3:40:34
22:50	47:46	1:45:50	3:42:12
23:00	48:07	1:46:36	3:43:49
23:10	48:28	1:47:23	3:45:26
23:20	48:49	1:48:09	3:47:04
23:30	49:10	1:48:55	3:48:41
23:40	49:31	1:49:42	3:50:18

5K	10K	Half-Marathon	Marathon
23:50	49:52	1:50:28	3:51:56
24:00	50:13	1:51:14	3:53:33
24:10	50:34	1:52:01	3:55:10
24:20	50:55	1:52:47	3:56:48
24:30	51:16	1:53:34	3:58:25
24:40	51:36	1:54:20	4:00:02
24:50	51:57	1:55:06	4:01:39
25:00	52:18	1:55:53	4:03:17
25:10	52:39	1:56:39	4:04:54
25:20	53:00	1:57:25	4:06:31
25:30	53:21	1:58:12	4:08:09
25:40	53:42	1:58:58	4:09:46
25:50	54:03	1:59:44	4:11:23
26:00	54:24	2:00:31	4:13:01
26:10	54:45	2:01:17	4:14:38
26:20	55:06	2:02:03	4:16:15
26:30	55:27	2:02:50	4:17:53
26:40	55:48	2:03:36	4:19:30
26:50	56:08	2:04:22	4:21:07
27:00	56:29	2:05:09	4:22:44
27:10	56:50	2:05:55	4:24:22
27:20	57:11	2:06:42	4:25:59
27:30	57:32	2:07:28	4:27:36
27:40	57:53	2:08:14	4:29:14
27:50	58:14	2:09:01	4:30:51
28:00	58:35	2:09:47	4:32:28
28:10	58:56	2:10:33	4:34:06
28:20	59:17	2:11:20	4:35:43
28:30	59:38	2:12:06	4:37:20
28:40	59:59	2:12:52	4:38:58
28:50	1:00:20	2:13:39	4:40:35
29:00	1:00:40	2:14:25	4:42:12
29:10	1:01:01	2:15:11	4:43:50
29:20	1:01:22	2:15:58	4:45:27

5K	10K	Half-Marathon	Marathon
29:30	1:01:43	2:16:44	4:47:04
29:40	1:02:04	2:17:30	4:48:41
29:50	1:02:25	2:18:17	4:50:19
30:00	1:02:46	2:19:03	4:51:56
30:10	1:03:07	2:19:49	4:53:33
30:20	1:03:28	2:20:36	4:55:11
30:30	1:03:49	2:21:22	4:56:48
30:40	1:04:10	2:22:09	4:58:25
30:50	1:04:31	2:22:55	5:00:03
31:00	1:04:52	2:23:41	5:01:40
31:10	1:05:12	2:24:28	5:03:17
31:20	1:05:33	2:25:14	5:04:55
31:30	1:05:54	2:26:00	5:06:32
31:40	1:06:15	2:26:47	5:08:09
31:50	1:06:36	2:27:33	5:09:47
32:00	1:06:57	2:28:19	5:11:24
32:10	1:07:18	2:29:06	5:13:01
32:20	1:07:39	2:29:52	5:14:38
32:30	1:08:00	2:30:38	5:16:16
32:40	1:08:21	2:31:25	5:17:53
32:50	1:08:42	2:32:11	5:19:30
33:00	1:09:03	2:32:57	5:21:08
33:10	1:09:23	2:33:44	5:22:45
33:20	1:09:44	2:34:30	5:24:22
33:30	1:10:05	2:35:16	5:26:00
33:40	1:10:26	2:36:03	5:27:37
33:50	1:10:47	2:36:49	5:29:14
34:00	1:11:08	2:37:36	5:30:52
34:10	1:11:29	2:38:22	5:32:29
34:20	1:11:50	2:39:08	5:34:06
34:30	1:12:11	2:39:55	5:35:44
34:40	1:12:32	2:40:41	5:37:21
34:50	1:12:53	2:41:27	5:38:58
35:00	1:13:14	2:42:14	5:40:35

5K	10K	Half-Marathon	Marathon
35:10	1:13:35	2:43:00	5:42:13
35:20	1:13:55	2:43:46	5:43:50
35:30	1:14:16	2:44:33	5:45:27
35:40	1:14:37	2:45:19	5:47:05
35:50	1:14:58	2:46:05	5:48:42
36:00	1:15:19	2:46:52	5:50:19
36:10	1:15:40	2:47:38	5:51:57
36:20	1:16:01	2:48:24	5:53:34
36:30	1:16:22	2:49:11	5:55:11
36:40	1:16:43	2:49:57	5:56:49
36:50	1:17:04	2:50:43	5:58:26
37:00	1:17:25	2:51:30	6:00:03
37:10	1:17:46	2:52:16	6:01:41
37:20	1:18:07	2:53:03	6:03:18
37:30	1:18:27	2:53:49	6:04:55
37:40	1:18:48	2:54:35	6:06:32
37:50	1:19:09	2:55:22	6:08:10
38:00	1:19:30	2:56:08	6:09:47
38:10	1:19:51	2:56:54	6:11:24
38:20	1:20:12	2:57:41	6:13:02
38:30	1:20:33	2:58:27	6:14:39
38:40	1:20:54	2:59:13	6:16:16
38:50	1:21:15	3:00:00	6:17:54
39:00	1:21:36	3:00:46	6:19:31
39:10	1:21:57	3:01:32	6:21:08
39:20	1:22:18	3:02:19	6:22:46
39:30	1:22:39	3:03:05	6:24:23
39:40	1:22:59	3:03:51	6:26:00
39:50	1:23:20	3:04:38	6:27:37
40:00	1:23:41	3:05:24	6:29:15

REAL RUNNER REPORT

Hi Bill & Scott,

Hopefully, you never tire of hearing about the personal triumphs that people have achieved through your book *Run Less Run Faster*.

I am 51 years old and six months ago would not have described myself as a runner, but perhaps a sporadic and occasional "jogger" for cross-training only. My main sport was squash if you'd asked me then. To that point I had never raced other than Grade 9–10 high school cross-country meets, and my idea of a really long run was 10K.

Early this spring I got inspired to take on a "big goal" this year as a means to find a renewed interest in my overall fitness, and a marathon ultimately seemed like the right fit. But I knew literally nothing about how to train, what a realistic finish time would be to train for, nor what my body and mind together could accomplish. And I wanted to go about it all entirely on my own.

An acquaintance recommended your book. I read it, it made practical sense to me, and so I applied it to prepare for the Toronto Waterfront Marathon this past Sunday.

My goal was a 3:45 finish, which felt like an aggressive goal for a first marathon, but I felt it was possibly achievable, based on my training, so I went for it.

Well, my chip time on Sunday was 3:45:45. My splits were very consistent throughout and I was able to increase my pace for the last 3km and finish strongly. What an incredible feeling!

I am overjoyed that it went so well and have you both to thank.

Perhaps more importantly, I have found a completely new appreciation for running and the joys of training with purpose.

So, in short, thank you for imparting such usable advice and helping me gain a newfound love of running.

It sure worked for me and I'll continue to apply it for my continued pursuits.

All the best,

Brad McCamus
Management Consultant
Toronto, Canada

4

FIRST Steps for New Runners

Can FIRST programs be used by the brand-new runner? Absolutely. As long as you don't try to run too often, too long, or too fast too soon. We want new runners to enjoy their activity and keep enjoying it for a long time. That requires progressing slowly and not becoming a running dropout because of burnout, overtraining, or injury.

Injury, in particular, is common among novices because they are motivated and excited to go farther and faster. That zeal is reinforced because the gains as you begin an exercise program are significant. Those big gains encourage you to do more and more. We point out to beginners that small gains that seem subtle from day to day become dramatic over several months and years. We encourage all new runners to develop a solid base before tackling lofty goals, such as marathons. Use this book to help pace yourself.

We regularly hear from new runners who have never run a race of any distance, and they often ask whether we have a marathon schedule for the new runner. Frequently, the person who contacts us is hoping to run a marathon in the next six months. While it is possible to survive the marathon distance by walking and running, we advise against attempting such a challenge without adequate preparation. Start with a 5K or a 10K. It is much more enjoyable and healthier to train properly and still satisfy some reasonable intermediate goals prior to attempting the challenge of 26.2 miles.

In this chapter, you will find beginning-runner training programs that progress conservatively, starting with a combination of walking and running. Follow the programs as designed, even if the steps feel too easy at first. Your body needs to adapt to the new stresses associated with running. Even if your cardiorespiratory system is not being stressed, the anatomical structures may be overtaxed and weakened, due to your newfound activity. Gradually building a solid base from which to progress will ensure safe training and positive movement toward your goals.

At some point, your progress may become interrupted from fatigue. Pay attention to your body and recognize the signs of prolonged fatigue. Individuals vary considerably in how much training they can tolerate. Know your threshold of training. Insert a rest and recovery day regularly to keep from doing too much and becoming overtrained. Sometimes it takes more than a day—it might take a very easy training week.

Many who decide to start running do so as a way to lose weight. Be careful if you are carrying extra body weight, because running is a weight-bearing activity and extra pounds add stress to the joints, muscles, bones, and connective tissue. Non–weight-bearing cross-training is especially valuable for losing weight without elevating your risk of injury (see Chapter 7).

||||||

A COACH'S REPORT

Frankie Painter, a personal trainer in Deland, Florida, shared with us her success using the FIRST Novice 5K Program with her clients. Frankie reported that she has a 100% success rate with getting beginning runners to complete a 5K in 12 weeks, following the training program in Table 4.1. She said that "No one has ever tried it and not liked it." Frankie said the fact that the program is based on time and not speed is very important to them. In addition to following the Novice Program, she stresses the importance of the stretches and strength exercises found in Chapters 14 and 15. She reported that some of her clients progressed to the 5K Intermediate Training Program in Table 4.2 and even the more advanced program in Table 6.1. Below is a report that Frankie forwarded to FIRST from one of her clients, Donna Nassick.

For years I watched runners as they ran—through my neighborhood, on the beach, or throughout the park. They all made it look so easy. Oh, how I wished that I had that sort of determination, discipline, and stamina. I tried once or twice. Got up in the morning deciding to give it a try . . . how hard could it be? I would run for as long as I could, then practically collapse with my heart feeling like it would pop out of my chest. I just knew I would never be a runner.

Then one day I heard about a run/walk program that was being offered, with the goal being a 5K. I put the thought of it aside. How could I possibly start to run? After all, I was now 48 years old! But my interest was piqued. I went to the information session to see what it was all about. The trainer, Frankie, made us believe that it was possible with the FIRST run/walk program, so I signed up.

After the first couple of weeks I could not believe I was running a half a mile . . . without stopping!!! Then the half-mile turned into a mile, then two miles. How did running such short distances in the beginning turn into miles? As the weeks went by, and I got closer to my goal, I knew that there was no other way that I could have accomplished it without the run/walk program and the motivation from my trainer. I am thankful for both.

I did run my goal race, 3.1 miles, without stopping! You would have thought I had run a marathon! I was that happy!!

Donna Nassick

UPDATE

Frankie recently updated us, stating that everything in this "Coach's Report" still holds true. That is, she has had a 100% success rate with getting beginning runners to complete a 5K in 12 weeks, following the 5K Novice Training Program in Table 4.1.

Frankie wrote that through all the years she has coached new runners, the things they like and appreciate most about the FIRST program are that it's only three days per week and the runs are based on time, not pace. She said it seems that new runners are most scared to join a group if they think they will be the slowest, but this program takes that fear away.

She added, "Every single person who uses the program discovers that their goal is not only possible, but achievable." Frankie reported that she continues to teach a dynamic warm-up, along with stretches afterward, as well as encouraging strength training and cross-training on nonrunning days. "These components of the FIRST program have kept me healthy, which is why I stress them to my clients."

Becoming a Runner: Q & A

Q. *How do I get started?*

A. First, make sure that you don't have any health problems or injuries that would prevent you from starting an exercise program. If you have any existing medical problem or if you are over 40 years of age, we recommend that you get clearance from your physician before beginning an exercise program.

Q. *What about shoes?*

A. Get proper shoes and clothing for exercise. There are many good running shoes available, each with different features. Find someone who is knowledgeable about running shoes to assist you in choosing a shoe that fits you properly. You can usually find knowledgeable sales assistance at running specialty stores. Try visiting several running specialty stores. It will take only two or three visits before you see trends in recommendations.

Q. *When and where should I run?*

A. Whether you run in the morning, at noon, or in the evening is largely a personal preference. Be realistic in deciding what regular schedule you are most likely to follow consistently. You don't have to work out at the same time each day. Plan ahead and consider your other obligations. Schedule a time for your run and consider that an important personal priority. Consistency is essential in establishing a habit.

Choose a place that is safe to run. A running track is a good place to start. Preferably, run in daylight. If you must run in the dark, choose a place that is well-lit. You must be mindful of safety and security. Many runners have sprained an ankle stepping off the curb in the dark. It may be a good idea to invest in some reflective gear while you're at the running specialty store.

Q. *How much should I do at first?*

A. FIRST has developed three 12-week programs that progress very gradually. Follow these programs carefully and you will enjoy the benefits of improved fitness and health, along with the exhilaration of completing a 5K race. It's important that you don't try to do too much too soon. It's equally as important for you to be faithful to the program and establish consistency in your training.

If you have done some running in the past or you regularly play other sports—basketball, tennis, cycling, etc.—and are not overweight, you may be able to begin with the 5K Intermediate Training Program (Table 4.2) rather than the 5K Novice Training Program (Table 4.1). The novice program is for someone who has been inactive and is just beginning to exercise.

Q. *What if I am overweight?*

A. The FIRST running programs are not designed as weight-management programs. However, regular physical activity expends energy and can assist you in weight loss. You must also be mindful that excess weight can be stressful to your joints and connective tissue. Combining a sensible diet with exercise is the safest and most effective way to reach a healthier weight.

If you are more than 30 pounds overweight, walking rather than running is advisable until you have lost your excess weight. To help reduce stress on your joints, cross-training on non–weight-bearing exercise machines is also recommended until you have lost your excess weight.

Q. *Should I get a partner to train with or join a group?*

A. *Yes!* Research shows clearly that compliance with an exercise schedule is better for those who have a training partner or who are part of a group that meets regularly to train. The commitment to others appears to be a powerful motivator.

Q. *Why does FIRST recommend starting with a 5K? Many people are joining marathon training groups, even though they have no running experience.*

A. FIRST believes that you need to establish a solid fitness base gradually before attempting a long race too soon; that can result in an injury. The exhilaration of running a 5K can be equal to or better than that of walking and running a longer race.

As health educators, we are interested in promoting running as a healthy, lifelong physical activity. Progressing gradually and developing the fitness and endurance for a 5K before moving on to a 10K, a half-marathon, or a marathon is a healthy approach. The physiological development for running peaks after about 8 to 10 years of training. Why not tackle these longer races when you are better prepared physically to do so?

You will have a much better running experience at these longer distances by running shorter races first. Many people join a charity training group without any running experience and complete the longer race—half-marathon or marathon—in survival mode. FIRST wants runners fully prepared for the race distance that they attempt.

Q. *As a novice, can I use any of the rest of this book?*

A. Yes, once you complete the 5K Novice Training Program (Table 4.1) and complete your first 5K, then you can refer to the paces provided in the tables for the intermediate program (Table 4.2). After completing the 5K Intermediate Training Program, then you will be ready to use the 5K Training Program (Table 6.1) found in Chapter 6.

TABLE 4.1

5K NOVICE TRAINING PROGRAM

The 5K Novice Training Program is designed to gradually move the inactive individual from walker to runner. It begins primarily with walking, interspersed with short intervals of running during a half-hour workout. Workout #1 in Week 12 includes walking for 10 minutes. Following that 10 minutes of walking, you will run for 1 minute and then walk for 2 minutes, which will be repeated four times. After completing the fourth repetition of 1-minute running and two minutes of walking, walk for 10 minutes. Run at a comfortable pace. Metric distances appear in italics.

W=Walk R=Run

WEEK	WORKOUT #1	WORKOUT #2	WORKOUT #3
12	32 total minutes: W: 10 min (R: 1 min, W: 2 min) x 4 W: 10 min	32 total minutes: W: 10 min (R: 1 min, W: 2 min) x 4 W: 10 min	32 total minutes: W: 10 min (R: 1 min, W: 2 min) x 4 W: 10 min
11	32 total minutes: W: 10 min (R: 2 min, W: 2 min) x 3 W: 10 min	32 total minutes: W: 10 min (R: 2 min, W: 2 min) x 3 W: 10 min	32 total minutes: W: 10 min (R: 2 min, W: 2 min) x 3 W: 10 min
10	32 total minutes: W: 10 min (R: 2 min, W: 1 min) x 4 W: 10 min	32 total minutes: W: 10 min (R: 2 min, W: 1 min) x 4 W: 10 min	35 total minutes: W: 10 min (R: 3 min, W: 2 min) x 3 W: 10 min
9	36 total minutes: W: 10 min (R: 3 min, W: 1 min) x 4 W: 10 min	36 total minutes: W: 10 min (R: 3 min, W: 1 min) x 4 W: 10 min	40 total minutes: W: 10 min (R: 3 min, W: 1 min) x 5 W: 10 min
8	44 total minutes: W: 10 min (R: 4 min, W: 2 min) x 4 W: 10 min	44 total minutes: W: 10 min (R: 4 min, W: 2 min) x 4 W: 10 min	45 total minutes: W: 10 min (R: 4 min, W: 1 min) x 5 W: 10 min

WEEK	WORKOUT #1	WORKOUT #2	WORKOUT #3
7	50 total minutes: W: 10 min (R: 4 min, W: 1 min) x 6 W: 10 min	50 total minutes: W: 10 min (R: 4 min, W: 1 min) x 6 W: 10 min	50 total minutes: W: 10 min (R: 5 min, W: 1 min) x 5 W: 10 min
6	56 total minutes: W: 10 min (R: 5 min, W: 1 min) x 6 W: 10 min	56 total minutes: W: 10 min (R: 5 min, W: 1 min) x 6 W: 10 min	55 total minutes: W: 10 min (R: 6 min, W: 1 min) x 5 W: 10 min
5	~50 total minutes: W: 10 min R: 1 mile (*1.5K*) W: 5 min (R: 6 min, W: 1 min) x 3 W: 10 min	~50 total minutes: W: 10 min R: 1 mile (*1.5K*) W: 5 min (R: 6 min, W: 1 min) x 3 W: 10 min	~45 total minutes: W: 10 min R: 1 mile (*1.5K*) W: 5 min R: 1 mile (*1.5K*) W: 10 min
4	~35 total minutes: W: 10 min R: 1.5 miles (*2K*) W: 10 min	~40 total minutes: W: 10 min R: 1.5 miles (*2K*) W: 5 min R: .5 mile (*1K*) W: 5 min	~35 total minutes: W: 10 min R: 2 miles (*3K*) W: 5 min
3	~35 total minutes: W: 10 min R: 2 miles (*3K*) W: 5 min	~35 total minutes: W: 10 min R: 2 miles (*3K*) W: 5 min	~40 total minutes: W: 10 min R: 2.5 miles (*4K*) W: 5 min
2	~40 total minutes: W: 10 min R: 2 miles (*3K*) W: 10 min	~40 total minutes: W: 10 min R: 2 miles (*3K*) W: 10 min	~45 total minutes: W: 10 min R: 3 miles (*5K*) W: 5 min
1	~40 total minutes W: 10 min R: 2 miles (*3K*) W: 10 min	~40 total minutes: W: 10 min R: 2 miles (*3K*) W: 10 min	~45 total minutes: W: 10 min R: 3.1 miles (*5K*) Race W: 5 min

TABLE 4.2

5K INTERMEDIATE TRAINING PROGRAM

This training schedule is for the runner who has completed the 5K Novice Training Program or who can run 5 kilometers. The workouts include the basic FIRST Key Runs described in Chapter 6. The paces for the Intermediate Program can be found in Chapter 6 (Tables 6.6 and 6.7).

RI = Recovery Interval of 400-meter walk/jog after each repeat.

Metric equivalents appear in italics.

WEEK	KEY RUN #1	KEY RUN #2	KEY RUN #3
12	10-min warm-up run 2 x 400 (RI) 10-min cool-down run	1 mile (*1.5km*) warm-up run 1 mile (*1.5km*) short tempo 1 mile (*1.5km*) cool-down run	3 miles (*5km*) @ mid-tempo pace
11	10-min warm-up run 3 x 400 (RI) 10-min cool-down run	1 mile (*1.5km*) warm-up run 1 mile (*1.5km*) short tempo 1 mile (*1.5km*) cool-down run	3 miles (*5km*) @ mid-tempo pace
10	10-min warm-up run 4 x 400 (RI) 10-min cool-down run	1 mile (*1.5km*) warm-up run 1 mile (*1.5km*) short tempo 1 mile (*1.5km*) cool-down run	3.5 miles (*6km*) @ mid-tempo pace
9	10-min warm-up run 2 x 400, 1 x 800 (RI) 10-min cool-down run	1 mile (*1.5km*) warm-up run 1.5 miles (*2km*) short tempo 1 mile (*1.5km*) cool-down run	3.5 miles (*6km*) @ mid-tempo pace
8	10-min warm-up run 400, 600, 800 (RI) 10-min cool-down run	1 mile (*1.5km*) warm-up run 1.5 miles (*2km*) short tempo 1 mile (*1.5km*) cool-down run	4 miles (*7km*) @ mid-tempo pace

WEEK	KEY RUN #1	KEY RUN #2	KEY RUN #3
7	10-min warm-up run 5 x 400 (RI) 10-min cool-down run	1 mile (*1.5km*) warm-up run 1 mile (*1.5km*) short tempo 1 mile (*1.5km*) cool-down run	4 miles (*7km*) @ mid-tempo pace
6	10-min warm-up run 400, 2 x 800 (RI) 10-min cool-down run	1 mile (*1.5km*) warm-up run 1.5 miles (*2km*) short tempo 1 mile (*1.5km*) cool-down run	4.5 miles (*7.5km*) @ mid-tempo pace
5	10-min warm-up run 2 x 1000 (RI) 10-min cool-down run	1 mile (*1.5km*) warm-up run 2 miles (*3km*) short tempo 1 mile (*1.5km*) cool-down run	4.5 miles (*7.5km*) @ mid-tempo pace
4	10-min warm-up run 6 x 400 (RI) 10-min cool-down run	1 mile (*1.5km*) warm-up run 2 miles (*3km*) short tempo 1 mile (*1.5km*) cool-down run	5 miles (*8km*) @ long-tempo pace
3	10-min warm-up run 3 x 800 (RI) 10-min cool-down run	1 mile (*1.5km*) warm-up run 2 miles (*3km*) short tempo 1 mile (*1.5km*) cool-down run	5 miles (*8km*) @ long-tempo pace
2	10-min warm-up run 200, 400, 600, 800 (RI) 10-min cool-down run	1 mile (*1.5km*) warm-up run 2 miles (*3km*) short tempo 1 mile (*1.5km*) cool-down run	5 miles (*8km*) @ long-tempo pace
1	10-min warm-up run 4 x 400 (RI) 10-min cool-down run	2 miles (*3km*) Easy 10-min walk	5K Race

REAL RUNNER REPORT

Good Afternoon, Coaches!

I wanted to send you an email of praise for your FIRST method for marathon training. I started running marathons in 2012 after saying that I would never do it. I fell in love with the challenge and preparation, and have been hooked ever since. I had boy/girl twins in 2010 and had been a runner, albeit not fast or competitive, for several years before. I had run a few halfs and never really tried to "race" them. When I took on the marathon challenge, I joined a group of FAST people who never ran without a plan. This was news to me, as I was your typical throw-on-some-shoes-and-go gal. After training with this group, having no idea about splits, tempo, and intervals, but rather just following along, I realized that I was actually pretty fast when properly trained—I completed my first race and qualified for BOSTON with a 3:21:23!

After qualifying and registering for Boston, I began to think that there is no way I can run the Super Bowl of races having only completed one marathon, so I bought your book and drafted a plan of my own. I started training to run in between marathons for experience and to see if I could go "low" with some real planning. I also realized through the process that my body was not equipped with the ability to run hard every day and it reminded me of that with a nagging IT band injury. Your three-quality-runs plan was the perfect solution while I trained and nursed my IT band back to health with swimming and PT.

I have now completed five marathons to include Boston 3:26, Chicago 3:23 (while evacuated from Savannah with my whole family for a hurricane), Marine Corps 3:15, and Savannah 3:21 and 3:16! In the years in between, your plan has helped me regain my speed after another pregnancy in 2015. I am currently training for the NYC marathon and hoping to have another PR.

Thanks,

Ashley Glover
CEO, Core Enthusiast, LLC
Savannah, Georgia

AN UPDATE ────────────────────────────────

Hello again, Bill,

I raced New York last fall with 3:16:55 and Boston in April 3:16 as well!

██████████████████████████████████████ IIIIII

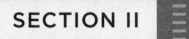

BECOMING FASTER WITH FIRST

5

FIRST Fundamentals

To benefit fully from the FIRST 3Plus2 Training Program, you need to perform all five workouts each week. The cumulative training effect of the workouts over 12 to 16 weeks translates into improved cardiorespiratory fitness, faster running, and improved endurance. We have learned that most runners do not focus on speed and running faster; their workouts lack variety; they do not allow for sufficient recovery; and they do not realize the value of cross-training.

We also hear from runners using our program that once they begin to follow a FIRST Training Program, they find the training paces challenging, but, surprisingly, with a focused effort and adequate recovery, are able to run the target times/paces. The FIRST Training Program is designed to take runners gradually to more demanding workouts. The gradual progression of stress and overload stimulates improvement in the cardiorespiratory system and muscle tissue responsible for running performance.

In addition to the three Key Runs per week described in Chapter 6, an integral part of the 3Plus2 Training Program is the aerobic cross-training. The "plus2" aspect of the training program includes at least two cross-training workouts each week. In Chapter 7, there are descriptions of specific cross-training workouts that complement the three key running workouts. You may choose from among the different cross-training workouts those you wish to use to supplement your running. While the FIRST 3Plus2 Training Program reduces the amount of running that you do weekly, it does not limit your cardiorespiratory training to three days a week. There has been a misconception by some runners that the FIRST Training Program is only three training days per week. The total training volume of the FIRST 3Plus2 Training Program includes three key running workouts and a minimum of two key cross-training workouts. So while it may be *running* less, the 3plus2 program is not *training* less.

Is it possible to be fit and race successfully by completing the three Key Runs without doing the cross-training? By this point in the book, you know that we believe strongly the cross-training is valuable and essential for optimal fitness and performance.

As runners, we are well aware that stretching, strength training, and form drills are typically neglected by most runners. Runners assume that more time spent running will be more beneficial than devoting some of their limited time and energy to these supplemental training exercises. Successful endurance performance is more than just running. If runners would devote time to these often overlooked, but important aspects of their preparation, their running would improve. However, once those same runners are injured, they spend much of their rehabilitation time cross-training, strength training, and stretching, all components of the FIRST training approach.

In keeping with our philosophy of getting the optimal benefits from a minimal time commitment, we have selected what we consider the most essential strength-training exercises (Chapter 14) and stretches (Chapter 15) for performance enhancement and injury prevention to include in your program. In Chapter 16, we show how to efficiently bring it all together—the three Key Runs, two cross-training workouts, strength training, and stretching exercises—to complete the FIRST Training Program in a minimum of seven hours per week.

Often, runners, in their zeal to get faster, engage in risky training that may not contribute to being healthier. Through repetition, many runners will incur overuse injuries and create muscular imbalances. We want to promote a fitter and healthier runner, not just a faster one. Smart training can help the runner be faster, fitter, and healthier. Chapters 6 and 7 provide the essentials of the aerobic component of the FIRST Training Program, designed to promote faster running, while contributing to your overall health and prolonging your running career. The information in the later chapters about stretching, strength training, recovery, year-round training, and nutrition are essential for producing a well-balanced runner.

How to Start Using the Training Programs

All the training target times and paces for all the Key Runs in the next chapter are based on your current running fitness level as represented by your most recent 5K race time or an estimate of your 5K race time. If you have a recent 5K race finish time that is representative of your current running fitness level, use it for selecting your target times from Table 6.6 and for determining your training paces from Tables 6.7 and 6.8. If you do not have a 5K time that reflects your current fitness, but you have a recent 10K time that is indicative of your current fitness, use Table 3.1 and find the 5K time equivalent to your 10K time and use it for selecting target times and paces from Tables 6.6–6.8.

If you do not have a 5K or 10K race finish time that represents your current fitness level, go to a 400-meter track and, after a good warm-up (e.g., 1–1.5 mile jog or 10–15 minutes of easy jogging), run 3 x 1600 meters (four laps around the track) with one-minute recovery between each 1600-meter run. During the one-minute recovery, you can walk around, but don't jog. Try to run the fastest time that you can maintain for all three 1600 meters. The goal is to have little variation in the times for the three 1600s.

||||||

TWO EXAMPLES OF USING 3 X 1600M FOR ESTIMATING YOUR 5K RACE TIME

EXAMPLE 1:

First 1600m:	7:05	(One-minute recovery)
Second 1600m:	7:15	(One-minute recovery)
Third 1600m:	7:40	
Average 1600m:	7:20	

EXAMPLE 2: First 1600m: 7:15 (One-minute recovery)

                Second 1600m: 7:20 (One-minute recovery)

                Third 1600m: 7:25

                Average 1600m: 7:20

In both of the 3 x 1600m workout examples, the average time for the 3 x 1600 meters with one-minute recovery was 7:20. After adding 15 seconds to the average time, both would indicate a 7:35 predicted 5K race pace. However, the first example had too much variation in the 1600s for it to be a valid estimate of the runner's 5K time. We would recommend that the runner in Example 1 redo the workout. It's very likely that the result of another set of 3 x 1600m with a smaller variation in the repeat times will be a better estimate of that runner's 5K race time.

After you have finished the 3 x 1600m run workout, average the time of the three 1600 repeats and add 15 seconds to the average for a prediction of your 5K per-mile race pace. For example, if your average 1600-meter time is 7:20, add 15 seconds and use 7:35 per mile as your predicted 5K race pace (which would be 23:34; see Appendix B).

To find your metric equivalent, multiply your average 1600-meter time by .62 and add 9 seconds. For example, if your average 1600-meter time is 8:00, multiply by .62, which equals 4.96 minutes, or 4:57.6. Add 9 seconds and use 5:06.6, or 5:07 per kilometer as your predicted 5K race pace (which would be 25:35; see Appendix B).

Now that you have an estimate of your current running fitness, as determined above, go to the pace tables in Appendix B and find your predicted 5K finish time. You will use that 5K time for selecting your training target times and paces for the three Key Runs in Chapter 6.

If you do not have a 5K or 10K race finish time that represents your current fitness level and you currently do not do any speed work—you only do distance running and you never run fast quarter-miles, half-miles, or miles—don't attempt to do the 3 x 1600-meter workout to determine your predicted 5K race time until you experience some speed training over the next two weeks.

In the first week, go to the track and do 4 x 800 meters with a 400-meter jog in between 800 repeats. Try to run a pace that you can maintain throughout the four-repeat workout. Check your times for each repeat. The purpose of this workout is to get accustomed to running faster than you normally run and to get a sense of pace for eventually performing the 3 x 1600 meter workout described in the previous section.

In the next week, go to the track and run 1 x 800 meters followed by a 400-meter jog recovery, followed by 1 x 1600 meters with a 400-meter jog recovery, and finish the workout with another 800 meters. Again, you should try to hold an even pace throughout the workout and record your times so that you have a sense of what you can maintain during the next week when you perform the 3 x 1600 meter workout to get your 5K predicted race time, which you'll use to select your training target times and paces from Tables 6.6 to 6.8.

In the first edition of this book, we indicated that you could use your half-marathon or marathon race finish times to predict your 5K race time by using Table 3.1. But we found that this approach is not the best predictor for many runners because it has become increasingly common for runners to race only half-marathons and marathons. Often, they do no speed training and their training is limited to long, slow runs. For that reason, their predicted 5K race time using Table 3.1 would not be a valid predictor of their 5K race performance. Simply put, they have focused only on endurance and not speed. Therefore, if you have raced only half-marathons and marathons and have not included speed training—track repeats/interval training—you need to follow the instructions in the previous section to determine your current 5K fitness level.

Why is having a current, valid 5K race time important? The three Key Runs of the FIRST Training Program all specify a target time or pace for each run workout. To get the full benefits from each run, you need to train at the appropriate intensity for producing a physiological adaptation that improves your running fitness. Thousands of runners have reported that the training targets based on their 5K race times remarkably match their abilities. The common phrase reported in their messages to us is that the training targets are "challenging, but doable." Once you determine the 5K race time that represents your current running fitness status, go to Chapter 6 and read about the three Key Runs.

Here is an example of a 3plus2 aerobic training week. It can be modified as long as the Key Runs are not completed on consecutive days. Chapter 6 describes in detail the three Key Runs and Chapter 7 describes the aerobic cross-training workouts. In Chapter 16, we describe how to add functional strength training and stretching to the cardiorespiratory training in the 7-Hour Workout Week.

THE 3plus2 TRAINING WEEK						
DAY 1	DAY 2	DAY 3	DAY 4	DAY 5	DAY 6	DAY 7
Cross-Train #1	Key Run #1	Cross-Train #2	Key Run #2	Off	Key Run #3	Cross-Train or Rest

DAY 1 **CROSS-TRAINING WORKOUT #1** (For 5K and 10K training, see Tables 7.1 and 7.2; for half-marathon and marathon training, see Tables 7.3 and 7.4.)

DAY 2 **KEY RUN #1: TRACK REPEATS** (See Tables 6.1–6.5 for training schedules and Table 6.6 for training target times.)

DAY 3 **CROSS-TRAINING WORKOUT #2** (For 5K and 10K training, see Tables 7.1 and 7.2; for half-marathon and marathon training, see Tables 7.3 and 7.4.)

DAY 4 **KEY RUN #2: TEMPO RUN** (See Tables 6.1–6.5 for training schedules and Table 6.7 for paces.)

DAY 5 **REST DAY**

DAY 6 **KEY RUN #3: LONG RUN** (See Tables 6.1–6.5 for training schedules and Table 6.8 for paces.)

DAY 7 **REST DAY** or **OPTIONAL CROSS-TRAINING**

Training for 5K, 10K, Half-Marathon, and Marathon

TRAINING FOR A 5K: Complete three Key Runs from Table 6.1 and two cross-training workouts from Tables 7.1 and 7.2. Times and paces for the Key Runs are in Tables 6.6–6.8.

TRAINING FOR A 10K: Complete three Key Runs from Table 6.2 and two cross-training workouts from Tables 7.1 and 7.2. Times and paces for the Key Runs are in Tables 6.6–6.8.

TRAINING FOR A HALF-MARATHON: Complete three Key Runs from Table 6.3 and two cross-training workouts from Tables 7.3 and 7.4. Times and paces for the Key Runs are in Tables 6.6–6.8.

TRAINING FOR A MARATHON: Complete three Key Runs from either Table 6.4 or Table 6.5 and two cross-training workouts from Tables 7.3 and 7.4. Times and paces for the Key Runs are in Tables 6.6–6.8.

||||||

REAL RUNNER REPORT

Hiya!

I'm a diehard FIRST convert. I bought your book and switched to your training plan after 11 unsuccessful attempts to qualify for Boston. I qualified and have since dropped my time by several more minutes. THANK YOU!

Here's my question: I ran a marathon (a PR!) and I'd like to do a 50-miler. It'll be my first ultra. I am wondering if I can make the FIRST program work for my situation. I don't want to lose my marathon base training and have to start from scratch, but I also don't know if it's wise to try to maintain this level for six straight months. Can you recommend a three-day-per-week program to get me through to a 50-miler?

Thank you SO much! For everything!

Ellen Hunter Gans
Writer
Edina, Minnesota

Bill and Scott,

I owe you a huge debt of gratitude. You were the first people to suggest that, even after 16 marathons, I could feasibly break 3:30. Per this email thread, you encouraged me to keep trying to get faster in "shorter" distances (e.g., marathon and below) before I switched to ultra distances.

You were right. I thought last fall's 3:30:07, referenced above, was my limit. I ran marathon number #17 in March, using your program, and ran a 3:23:30. I then thought THAT was my limit.

I ran marathon #18 yesterday—the same course at which I ran the 3:30:07 in 2016—and ran a 3:17:07.

Before trying the FIRST program, I was stalled at around 4:12. I've since cut nearly an hour off that time.

Thank you. Thank you. Thank you. You took a lifelong junior varsity athlete and made her into a quasi-respectable marathoner at age 34. (But seriously, I think I'm maxed out now. :-))

6

Three Quality Runs

The "3" of the 3Plus2 Training Program

"I was skeptical when I started your training program, but I found that the challenging, but doable, run workouts caused me to get stronger and faster week after week." That's the most common refrain from readers who train using the FIRST Training Programs. The three-runs-per-week training program defies conventional thinking about the necessity of piling on the training miles.

Most runners who incorporate the three quality runs that are a part of the FIRST method into their training find that their fitness improves, as do their race times. What explains this? Most runners focus on the frequency and duration of their training. Their conversations begin with "How many times did you run?" and end with "How many miles did you log this week?" They neglect the importance of intensity—the pace of each run workout. Try running the paces designated in the tables provided in this chapter and watch your race times improve.

While a certain fitness base is necessary, quality performances are determined more by intensity than by volume. Workouts that cause you to go really hard, recover, and go hard again have significant physiological benefits. Workouts that cause you to sustain a moderately hard effort for 20 to 30 minutes also train your body to exercise for long periods near your maximum effort. Doing long runs at speeds progressively closer to your marathon pace causes you to adapt to the stress of running hard for several hours to prepare for a marathon.

This chapter supplies you with the training paces appropriate for your current fitness level—paces that will lead to improvements in your fitness level and future running performances. The chapter also provides the nuts-and-bolts descriptions for your three quality runs per week, the heart of the 3Plus2 Training Program. You will find all the details necessary for performing the three weekly quality runs. Following the discussion of the overall design of the program are tables that show you how to determine your target time and pace for each run (see Tables 6.6–6.8) and the training schedules for 5K, 10K, half-marathon, and marathon races (see Tables 6.1–6.5). First, however, we present a brief discussion of the science underlying the FIRST program.

Three Quality Runs: The Science

The theoretical concept underlying the FIRST training regimen is that each run be performed with a goal of improving one of the primary physiological processes and running performance variables. The training programs are designed to help runners train effectively, efficiently and to avoid overtraining and injury.

Maximal Oxygen Consumption (VO_2 max) is a measure of the ability of an athlete to produce energy aerobically. You might say that maximal oxygen consumption gives a runner an idea of how large an engine he has to work with. Normally, a higher VO_2 max indicates that more work can be performed during a given time period. This simply means that an individual with a higher VO_2 max should be able to run faster than an otherwise comparable runner with a lower VO_2 max. A high maximal capacity to deliver oxygenated blood means there is the potential for more muscles to be active simultaneously during exercise. Values for VO_2 max typically range between 40 and 80 ml/kg/min (milliliters of oxygen per kilogram of body weight per minute). Research has shown VO_2 max to increase as much as 20% through a combination of endurance and interval training. VO_2 max and submaximal exercise capacities are limited by different mechanisms. VO_2 max appears to be related more to cardiovascular factors, such as maximal cardiac output, whereas skeletal muscle metabolic factors, including respiratory enzyme activity, play more of a role in determining submaximal exercise capacity.

Lactate Threshold (LT) is a measure of metabolic fitness. Lactate is an organic by-product of anaerobic metabolism, and its accumulation in the blood is used to evaluate the intensity that a runner can maintain for extended periods—usually 30 minutes or more. Lactate threshold and maximal steady state lactate levels are indications of how well your muscles are trained to do endurance-type work. Most people, except the most highly trained athletes, are limited by metabolic fitness rather than cardiovascular fitness. Highly trained endurance athletes can work at extreme heart rates without severe muscle fatigue. An untrained individual might reach LT at about 50–60% of her maximum heart rate, whereas a well-trained runner won't reach lactate threshold until about 80–95% of his maximum heart rate.

Running Economy is the amount of oxygen being consumed relative to the runner's body weight and running speed. Unnecessary body motion results in an increase in oxygen consumption and thus a decrease in running economy. Running economy can be expressed either as the velocity achieved for a given rate of oxygen consumption or the VO_2 necessary to maintain a given running speed. Running at a given submaximal pace and using less oxygen indicate that a runner is more economical or has improved her running economy. This determinant of running performance generally takes the longest period of training for measurable improvements.

Training at the appropriate intensity is generally recognized as the most important factor for improving each of the three elements. For that reason, each workout needs to have the appropriate intensity, or running pace, that stimulates the physiological adaptation needed for improving each of the three determinants of running performance.

Running speed is determined by stride length and stride frequency. Stride length is increased if there is more power available in the push-off phase of the gait, not in artificially trying to increase the stride by landing the foot out in front of the knee. Having more power comes from being stronger from the hips and lower extremities. Stride frequency can be improved by limiting the amount of ground contact time with each foot strike.

THREE QUALITY RUNS: THE ESSENTIALS

	Type of Training		
Elements	**Key Run #1** **Track Repeats**	**Key Run #2** **Tempo Run**	**Key Run #3** **Long Run**
Purpose	Improve VO$_2$ max, running speed, and running economy	Improve endurance by raising lactate threshold	Improve endurance by raising aerobic metabolism
Intensity	5K race pace or slightly faster	Comfortably hard; 15 to 45 sec slower than 5K race pace	Approximately 30 sec slower than goal marathon pace
Duration of run	10 min or less	20 to 45 min at tempo pace	60 to 180 min
Frequency	Repeat shorter segments until quality work totals about 5K per session	One tempo run per week	One long run per week

Key Run #1: Track Repeats or Interval Training

Warm-up

The warm-up for the Track Repeats is especially important because of the fast running to be performed. You do not want to start these repeated intervals of fast running without preparing the body for the intense activity.

A proper warm-up for Key Run #1 should include easy jogging, dynamic stretches, fast strides, and a couple of drills. Below is a description of the warm-up sequence.

1. Start with 10–15 minutes of easy jogging.

2. Perform the dynamic stretches shown in Chapter 15 (takes 5 minutes).

3. Perform two 100-meter strides. Strides are gradual accelerations for 80 meters until you reach approximately 90% of full speed with a deceleration over the final 20 meters. Recover for 30 seconds or less and repeat. Completion of the strides will make the initial track repeats much easier and reduce the shock of going from an easy warm-up jog to a near all-out effort on the repeats. Stay comfortable with the strides and focus on good form. You shouldn't be straining during the strides.

4. Perform two more 100-meter strides by doing "butt kicks" for 20 meters and then gradually accelerating for 60 meters and decelerating for 20 meters. Recover for 30 seconds, begin the next 100 meters and do "high knee lifts" for 20 meters, and then gradually accelerate for 60 meters and decelerate for 20 meters.

5. Now you are ready for Key Run #1.

The Track Repeats or Interval Training

Even though we refer to the interval training as "track repeats," the repeated intervals of fast running and recovery can be performed on any relatively flat terrain, not only on a track. Many runners like to perform them on trails with marked distances. Now that it is common to have a GPS watch that measures distance, the repeats can be done on the road or wherever there is a safe and relatively flat section of trail or road that is preferably 400 meters long.

The track repeats include running relatively short distances of 400 meters to 2000 meters, interspersed with brief recovery intervals on a repeated basis. Track repeats are designed to improve maximal oxygen consumption, running economy, and speed. Most of these workouts total about 5000 meters of fast running per session. Including warm-up and cool-down, Key Run #1 typically totals 5 to 6 miles or 8 to 10 kilometers.

Caution: Most runners can run the first few repeats faster than the specified target time. However, the goal is to run the entire workout at the target time with minimal deviation in the times for each repeat. Also, the objective is not to run the repeats as fast as you can; you have two other Key Runs to perform for the week; while track repeats are fast, they are not races. Do not sacrifice meeting the target times for the tempo and long runs by running the repeats at an exhausting speed that does not provide sufficient recovery for Key Runs #2 and #3.

Cool-down

After a challenging workout of repeats on the track, a cool-down is important. Jog slowly for 10–15 minutes.

Track Repeat Example 1: 6 x 800m (90 sec RI) means to repeat an 800-meter run six times, with a recovery interval of 90 seconds. In between the repeats, you recover by walking/jogging for 90 seconds. After the 90 seconds of recovery, you will start the next 800-meter run. The goal is to run all 800-meter runs at the same prescribed target time found in Table 6.6. Again, the goal of the workout is to keep a small range of times for the 800 meters. For example, rather than a set like 3:00, 2:58, 3:04, 3:08, 3:09, 3:02 (an 11-second range), shoot for a more consistent range of times, such as 3:02, 3:01, 3:02, 3:02, 3:03, 3:02 (a 2-second range). There should not be more than a couple of seconds' difference in your times for the repeats.

Track Repeat Example 2: 5 x 1km (400m RI) means five repeat runs of 1000 meters (2.5 times around a 400-meter track) with a 400-meter walk/jog as a recovery between repeat runs. Using your prescribed training pace for 1000 meters found in Table 6.6, try running the first repeat at the target time. Check your time after finishing the first repeat to make sure you aren't running too fast or not fast enough. Jog 400 meters at a relaxed and comfortable effort (for most people, this recovery lap will take 2 to 4 minutes) as your recovery. At the end of the jog recovery, begin the second repeat, concentrating on maintaining the prescribed pace. The times for running the five 1km repeats should vary no more than a few seconds.

The FIRST Training Program emphasizes to runners the importance of keeping a very small range of interval times for the entire workout. The target paces should be realistic and challenging, but not so difficult that you are unable to recover for Key Run #2. Our emphasis that the entire set of repeats be run within a range of only a couple of seconds pretty much ensures that you won't overdo it.

Key Run #2: Tempo Run

Warm-up

Begin with the dynamic stretches described in Chapter 15. They can be performed in 5 minutes.

Tempo runs begin with easy running for 1 or 2 miles (1.5–3km) prior to the faster tempo aspect of the workout. As with the strides on the track, the pace of the warm-up should gradually increase during the easy miles, so that you are close to tempo pace by the end of the warm-up.

Tempo portion

The tempo portion of the workout is typically 3 to 5 miles (5–8km) at 10K pace or slightly slower. For marathon training, the tempo portion is extended to 8 to 10 miles (13–16km) at your planned marathon pace.

Cool-down

A mile to 10 minutes of easy running is recommended for a cool-down after the tempo phase of the run.

Example: 1 mile (1.5km) warm-up, 2 miles (3km) at ST and 1 mile (1.5K) cool-down means to start slowly and gradually pick up the pace, and after one mile (1.5km), run the next two miles (3km) at the designated pace, based on your 5K race pace (see Table 6.7). This short-tempo pace (ST) is approximately 15 seconds slower than your per-mile 5K race pace and 9 seconds slower than your per-kilometer pace. After the 2-mile (3km) tempo effort, slow down and run an easy cool-down mile (1.5km). In this example, Key Run #2 is a continuous 4-mile or 6.5km run.

Key Run #3: Long Run

Warm-up

While there is not a specific warm-up for your long run, the early part of the long run can serve as the warm-up. The recommended long-run pace need not be achieved during the first couple of miles or kilometers.

Long run

The long run (relative to your goals and present training mileage) requires steady running from 6 to 20 miles (10–32km) at a pace equal to your 5K pace, plus 45 seconds for the 5K and 10K long runs. For the half-marathon and marathon long runs, the long-run pace is equal to your 5K pace, plus 75 to 90 seconds, or 15 to 30 seconds per mile or 9 to 19 seconds per kilometer slower than your planned marathon pace.

Try starting your training runs a bit slower than the prescribed pace and then pick up the pace in the middle section of your training run. Try to have a strong finish over the last couple of miles (kilometers) of your long training runs. Faster than recommended pace running during the middle phase of the long run can offset the earlier slower pace, so you can meet the average targeted pace for the entire run.

Cool-down

Ten minutes of easy walking after a long run serves as a good cool-down. Drinking a sports drink or a recovery drink during these 10 minutes will aid your recovery (see Chapter 8). Doing some of the basic static stretches described in Chapter 15 aids your recovery as well.

Example: 15 miles at MP + 30 means to run 15 miles 30 seconds per mile slower than your planned marathon pace. For a runner with a target marathon time of 3:10 or 7:15/mile pace, this long run might begin with a 7:55

mile, followed by a 7:50 mile, before settling into a 7:45/mile pace. After 5 miles of running at a 7:45/mile pace, you may want to try the next 3 or 4 miles at a 7:35–40 pace before running the last few miles at a 7:45/mile pace, or you may want to hold the 7:45/mile pace up through 12 miles and then try to run the last three miles faster than the 7:45/mile pace. You can alternate strategies from one long training run to the next. The metric version of this workout is 24km at MP + 19; this means you'll run 24 kilometers at 19 seconds per kilometer slower than your planned marathon pace. For a runner with a target marathon time of 3:10 or 4:30/kilometer pace, this long run might begin with a 4:55 pace, followed by a 4:45 kilometer before settling into a 4:49/kilometer pace. After 8 kilometers of running at a 4:49/kilometer pace, you may want to try the next 5 to 7 kilometers at a 4:40 to 4:45 pace before running the last few kilometers at a 4:49/kilometer pace, or you may want to hold the 4:49/kilometer pace up through 20km and then try to run the last 4km faster than a 4:49/kilometer pace.

Detailed Training Schedules for Four Popular Race Distances and Training

The FIRST 3Plus2 Training Programs for distances of 5K, 10K, half-marathon, novice marathon, and marathon follow in Tables 6.1 through 6.5. To find the appropriate training target time or pace for a specific distance, refer to Tables 6.6–6.8. If you have not run a 5K recently, refer to the description in Chapter 5 for determining target paces.

TABLE 6.1

5K Training Program: The Three Quality Runs

RI = Recovery Interval; which may be a timed recovery interval or a distance that you walk/jog.

Paces: ST—Short Tempo; MT—Mid Tempo; LT—Long Tempo. See Table 6.7.

Key Run #1 begins with a 10–20-min warm-up and ends with a 10-min cool-down. See Table 6.6 for target times.

Key Run #2 begins with a one-mile (1.5km) warm-up and ends with a one-mile (1.5km) cool-down. See Table 6.7.

Metric equivalents appear in bold italics.

WEEK	KEY RUN #1	KEY RUN #2	KEY RUN #3
12	8 x 400 (400 RI)	2 miles (*3km*) at ST	5 miles (*8km*) at LT
11	5 x 800 (400 RI)	3 miles (*5km*) at ST	6 miles (*10km*) at LT
10	2 x 1600 (400 RI) 1 x 800 (400 RI)	2 miles (*3km*) at ST 1 mile (*1.5km*) Easy 2 miles (*3km*) at ST	5 miles (*8km*) at LT
9	400, 600, 800, 800, 600, 400 (400 RI)	4 miles (*6.5km*) at MT	6 miles (*10km*) at LT
8	4 x 1000 (400 RI)	3 miles (*5km*) at ST	7 miles (*11km*) at LT
7	1600, 1200, 800, 400 (400 RI)	1 mile (*1.5km*) at ST 1 mile (*1.5km*) Easy 1 mile (*1.5km*) at ST 1 mile (*1.5km*) Easy 1 mile (*1.5km*) at ST	6 miles (*10km*) at LT
6	10 x 400 (90 sec RI)	4 miles (*7km*) at MT	8 miles (*13km*) at LT
5	6 x 800 (90 sec RI)	2 miles (*3km*) at ST 1 mile (*1.5km*) Easy 2 miles (*3km*) at ST	7 miles (*11km*) at LT

WEEK	KEY RUN #1	KEY RUN #2	KEY RUN #3
4	4 x 1200 (400 RI)	3 miles (*5km*) at ST	7 miles (*11km*) at LT
3	5 x 1000 (400 RI)	2 miles (*3km*) at ST 1 mile (*1.5km*) Easy 1 mile (*1.5km*) at ST 1 mile (*1.5km*) Easy 2 miles (*3km*) at ST	7 miles (*11km*) at LT
2	3 x 1600 (400 RI)	3 miles (*5km*) at ST	6 miles (*10km*) at LT
1	6 x 400 (60 sec RI)	3 miles (*5km*) Easy No additional warm-up or cool-down.	**5K Race**

TABLE 6.2

10K Training Program: The Three Quality Runs

RI = Recovery Interval; which may be a timed recovery interval or a distance that you walk/jog.

Paces: ST—Short Tempo; MT—Mid Tempo; LT—Long Tempo. See Table 6.7.

Key Run #1 begins with a 10–20-min warm-up and ends with a 10-min cool-down. See Table 6.6 for target times.

Key Run #2 begins with a one-mile (1.5km) warm-up and ends with a one-mile (1.5km) cool-down. See Table 6.7.

Metric equivalents appear in bold italics.

WEEK	KEY RUN #1	KEY RUN #2	KEY RUN #3
12	8 x 400 (400 RI)	3 miles (**5km**) at ST	6 miles (**10km**) at LT
11	5 x 800 (400 RI)	2 miles (**3km**) at ST 1 mile (**1.5km**) Easy 2 miles (**3km**) at ST	7 miles (**11km**) at LT
10	2 x 1600 (400 RI) 1 x 800 (400 RI)	4 miles (**7km**) at MT	8 miles (**13km**) at LT
9	400, 600, 800, 800, 600, 400 (400 RI)	2 miles (**3km**) at ST 1 mile (**1.5km**) Easy 1 mile (**1.5km**) at ST 1 mile (**1.5km**) Easy 2 miles (**3km**) at ST	9 miles (**14km**) at LT

WEEK	KEY RUN #1	KEY RUN #2	KEY RUN #3
8	4 x 1000 (400 RI)	4 miles (*7km*) at ST	10 miles (*16km*) at LT
7	1600, 1200, 800, 400 (400 RI)	5 Miles (*8km*) at MT	8 miles (*13km*) at LT
6	10 x 400 (90 sec RI)	3 miles (*5km*) at ST	10 miles (*16km*) at LT
5	6 x 800 (90 sec RI)	1 mile (*1.5km*) at ST 1 mile (*1.5km*) Easy 2 miles (*3km*) at ST 1 mile (*1.5km*) Easy 1 mile (*1.5km*) at ST	8 miles (*13km*) at LT
4	4 x 1200 (400 RI)	3 miles (*5km*) at ST	10 miles (*16km*) at LT
3	5 x 1000 (400 RI)	6 miles (*10km*) at MT	8 miles (*13km*) at LT
2	3 x 1600 (400 RI)	3 miles (*5km*) at ST	7 miles (*11km*) at LT
1	6 x 400 (60 sec RI)	3 miles (*5km*) Easy No additional warm-up or cool-down.	**10K Race**

TABLE 6.3

Half-Marathon Training Plan: The Three Quality Runs

RI = Recovery Interval; which may be a timed recovery interval or a distance that you walk/jog.

Paces: HMP—Half-Marathon Pace; ST—Short Tempo; MT—Mid Tempo; LT—Long Tempo. A plus sign (+) followed by a figure indicates seconds per mile or kilometer. See Tables 6.7–6.8.

Key Run #1 begins with a 10–20-min warm-up and ends with a 10-min cool-down. See Table 6.6 for target times.

Metric equivalents appear in bold italics.

WEEK	KEY RUN #1	KEY RUN #2	KEY RUN #3
16	12 x 400 (90 sec RI)	2 miles (*3km*) Easy 3 miles (*5km*) at ST 1 mile (*1.5km*) Easy	8 miles at HMP + 20 *13km at HMP + 13*
15	400, 600, 800, 1200, 800, 600, 400 (400 RI)	5 miles (*8km*) at MT 1 mile (*1.5km*) Easy	9 miles at HMP + 20 *14km at HMP + 13*
14	6 x 800 (90 sec RI)	2 miles (*3km*) Easy 3 miles (*5km*) at ST 1 mile (*1.5km*) Easy	10 miles Easy *16km Easy*
13	5 x 1000 (400 RI)	1 mile (*1.5km*) Easy 3 miles (*5km*) at ST 1 mile (*1.5km*) Easy	9 miles at HMP + 20 *14km at HMP + 13*
12	3 x 1600 (60 sec RI)	1 mile (*1.5km*) Easy 6 miles (*10km*) at LT 1 mile (*1.5km*) Easy	11 miles at HMP + 30 *18km at HMP + 19*
11	2 x 1200 (2 min RI) 4 x 800 (2 min RI)	1 mile (*1.5km*) Easy 2 miles (*3km*) at MT 1 mile (*1.5km*) Easy 2 miles (*3km*) at MT 1 mile (*1.5km*) Easy	10 miles at HMP + 20 *16km at HMP + 13*
10	6 x 800 (90 sec RI)	1 mile (*1.5km*) Easy 5 miles (*8km*) at MT 1 mile (*1.5km*) Easy	12 miles at HMP + 30 *19km at HMP + 19*

WEEK	KEY RUN #1	KEY RUN #2	KEY RUN #3
9	2 x (6 x 400) (90 sec RI) (2:30 RI between sets)	1 mile (*1.5km*) Easy 2 miles (*3km*) at MT 1 mile (*1.5km*) Easy 2 miles (*3km*) at MT 1 mile (*1.5km*) Easy	8 miles at HMP + 20 ***13km at HMP + 13***
8	2 x 1600 (60 sec RI) 2 x 800 (60 sec RI)	1 mile (*1.5km*) Easy 5 miles (*8km*) at MT 1 mile (*1.5km*) Easy	13 miles at HMP + 30 ***21km at HMP + 19***
7	4 x 1200 (2 min RI)	1 mile (*1.5km*) Easy 6 miles (*10km*) at MT 1 mile (*1.5km*) Easy	10 miles at HMP + 20 ***16km at HMP + 13***
6	1km, 2km, 1km, 1km (400 RI)	1 mile (*1.5km*) Easy 5 miles (*8km*) at MT 1 mile (*1.5km*) Easy	14 miles at HMP + 30 ***22km at HMP + 19***
5	3 x 1600 (400 RI)	6 miles (*10km*) Easy	10 miles at HMP + 20 ***16km at HMP + 13***
4	10 x 400 (400 RI)	1 mlle (*1.5km*) Easy 5 miles (*8km*) at MT 1 mile (*1.5km*) Easy	15 miles at HMP + 30 ***24km at HMP + 19***
3	2 x 1200 (2:00 RI) 4 x 800 (2:00 RI)	1 mile (*1.5km*) Easy 5 miles (*8km*) at MT 1 mile (*1.5km*) Easy	12 miles at HMP + 20 ***19km at HMP + 13***
2	5 x 1000 (400 RI)	2 miles (*3km*) Easy 3 miles (*5km*) at ST 1 mile (*1.5km*) Easy	8 miles at HMP + 20 ***13km at HMP + 13***
1	6 x 400 (400 RI)	3 miles (*5km*) Easy No additional warm-up or cool-down.	Half-Marathon 13.1 miles (***21.1K***)

TABLE 6.4

Novice Marathon Training Plan: The Three Quality Runs

RI = Recovery Interval; which may be a timed recovery interval or a distance that you walk/jog.

Paces: HMP—Half-Marathon Pace; ST—Short Tempo; MT—Mid Tempo; LT—Long Tempo. A plus sign (+) followed by a figure indicates seconds per mile or kilometer. See Tables 6.7–6.8.

Key Run #1 begins with a 10–20-min warm-up and ends with a 10-min cool-down. See Table 6.6 for target times.

Metric equivalents appear in bold italics.

WEEK	KEY RUN #1	KEY RUN #2	KEY RUN #3
16	3 x 1600 (400 RI)	2 miles (*3km*) Easy 2 miles (*3km*) at ST 2 miles (*3km*) Easy	8 miles at MP + 30 sec *13km at MP + 19*
15	4 x 800 (2 min RI)	1 mile (*1.5km*) Easy 5 miles (*8km*) at MP 1 mile (*1.5km*) Easy	9 miles at MP + 45 *14km at MP + 28*
14	1200, 1000, 800, 600, 400 (200 RI)	1 mile (*1.5km*) Easy 5 miles (*8km*) at LT 1 mile (*1.5km*) Easy	10 miles at MP + 45 *16km at MP + 28*
13	5 x 1000 (400 RI)	1 mile (*1.5km*) Easy 4 miles (*7km*) at MT 1 mile (*1.5km*) Easy	11 miles at MP + 45 *18km at MP + 28*
12	3 x 1600 (400 RI)	2 miles (*3km*) Easy 3 miles (*5km*) at ST 1 mile (*1.5km*) Easy	12 miles at MP + 45 *19km at MP + 28*
11	2 x 1200 (2 min RI) 4 x 800 (2 min RI)	1 mile (*1.5km*) Easy 5 miles (*8km*) at MT 1 mile (*1.5km*) Easy	14 miles at MP + 45 *22km at MP + 28*
10	6 x 800 (90 sec RI)	1 mile (*1.5km*) Easy 6 miles (*10km*) at LT 1 mile (*1.5km*) Easy	10 miles at MP + 15 *16km at MP + 9*

WEEK	KEY RUN #1	KEY RUN #2	KEY RUN #3
9	2 x (6 x 400) (90 sec RI) (2 min 30 sec RI between sets)	2 miles (*3km*) Easy 3 miles (*5km*) at ST 1 mile (*1.5km*) Easy	15 miles at MP + 30 *24km at MP + 19*
8	2 x 1600 (60 sec RI) 2 x 800 (60 sec RI)	1 mile (*1.5km*) Easy 4 miles (*7km*) at MT 1 mile (*1.5km*) Easy	16 miles at MP + 30 *26km at MP + 19*
7	4 x 1200 (2 min RI)	10 miles (*16km*) at MP	12 miles at MP + 20 *19km at MP + 12*
6	1km, 2km, 1km, 1km (400 RI)	1 mile (*1.5km*) Easy 5 miles (*8km*) at MP 1 mile (*1.5km*) Easy	18 miles at MP + 45 *29km at MP + 28*
5	3 x 1600 (400 RI)	10 miles (*16km*) at MP	13 miles at MP + 15 *21km at MP + 9*
4	10 x 400 (400 RI)	10-min warm-up 8 miles (*13km*) at MP 10-min cool-down	20 miles at MP + 30 *32km at MP +19*
3	8 x 800 (90 sec RI)	1 mile (*1.5km*) Easy 5 miles (*8km*) at MT 1 mile (*1.5km*) Easy	13 miles at MP *21km at MP*
2	5 x 1000 (400 RI)	2 miles (*3km*) Easy 3 miles (*5km*) at ST 1 mile (*1.5km*) Easy	8 miles at MP *13km at MP*
1	6 x 400 (400 RI)	10-min warm-up 3 miles (*5K*) at MP 10-min cool-down	Marathon 26.2 miles *42.2km at MP*

TABLE 6.5

Marathon Training Plan: The Three Quality Runs

RI = Recovery Interval; which may be a timed recovery interval or a distance that you walk/jog.

Paces: HMP—Half Marathon Pace; ST—Short Tempo; MT—Mid Tempo; LT—Long Tempo. A plus sign (+) followed by a figure indicates seconds per mile or kilometer. See Tables 6.7–6.8.

Key Run #1 begins with a 10–20-min warm-up and ends with a 10-min cool-down. See Table 6.6 for target times.

Metric equivalents appear in bold italics.

WEEK	KEY RUN #1	KEY RUN #2	KEY RUN #3
16	3 x 1600 (400 RI)	2 miles (*3km*) Easy 2 miles (*3km*) at ST 2 miles (*3km*) Easy	13 miles at MP + 30 *21km at MP + 19*
15	4 x 800 (2 min RI)	1 mile (*1.5km*) Easy 5 miles (*8km*) at MP 1 mile (*1.5km*) Easy	15 miles at MP + 45 *24km at MP + 28*
14	1200, 1000, 800, 600, 400 (200RI)	1 mile (*1.5km*) Easy 5 miles (*8km*) at LT 1 mile (*1.5km*) Easy	17 miles at MP + 45 *27km at MP + 28*
13	5 x 1000 (400 RI)	1 mile (*1.5km*) Easy 4 miles (*7km*) at MT 1 mile (*1.5km*) Easy	20 miles at MP + 60 *32km at MP + 37*
12	3 x 1600 (400 RI)	2 miles (*3km*) Easy 3 miles (*5km*) at ST 1 mile (*1.5km*) Easy	18 miles at MP + 45 *29km at MP + 28*
11	2 x 1200 (2 min RI) 4 x 800 (2 min RI)	1 mile (*1.5km*) Easy 5 miles (*8km*) at MT 1 mile (*1.5km*) Easy	20 miles at MP + 45 *32km at MP + 28*
10	6 x 800 (90 sec RI)	1 mile (*1.5km*) Easy 6 miles (*10km*) at LT 1 mile (*1.5km*) Easy	13 miles at MP + 15 *21km at MP + 9*

WEEK	KEY RUN #1	KEY RUN #2	KEY RUN #3
9	2 x (6x 400) (90 sec RI) (2 min 30 sec RI between sets)	2 miles (*3km*) Easy 3 miles (*5km*) at ST 1 mile (*1.5km*) Easy	18 miles at MP + 30 *29km at MP + 19*
8	2 x 1600 (60 sec RI) 2 x 800 (60 sec RI)	1 mile (*1.5km*) Easy 4 miles (*7km*) at MT 1 mile (*1.5km*) Easy	20 miles at MP + 30 *32km at MP + 19*
7	4 x 1200 (2 min RI)	10 miles (*16km*) at MP	15 miles at MP + 20 *24km at MP + 12*
6	1km, 2km, 1km, 1km (400 RI)	1 mile (*1.5km*) Easy 5 miles (*8km*) at MP 1 mile (*1.5km*) Easy	20 miles at MP + 30 *32km at MP + 19*
5	3 x 1600 (400 RI)	10 miles (*16km*) at MP	15 miles at MP + 15 *24km at MP + 9*
4	10 x 400 (400 RI)	10-min warm-up 8 miles (*13km*) at MP 10-min cool-down	20 miles at MP + 15 *32km at MP + 9*
3	8 x 800 (90 sec RI)	1 mile (*1.5km*) Easy 5 miles (*8km*) at MT 1 mile (*1.5km*) Easy	13 miles at MP *21km at MP*
2	5 x 1000 (400 RI)	2 miles (*3km*) Easy 3 miles (*5km*) at ST 1 mile (*1.5km*) Easy	10 miles at MP *16km at MP*
1	6 x 400 (400 RI)	10-min warm-up 3 miles (*5K*) at MP 10-min cool-down	Marathon 26.2 miles *42.2km at MP*

TABLE 6.6

Key Run #1 Target Times

(Improves economy, running speed, and VO₂ max)

5K-time	400m	600m	800m	1000m	1200m	1600m	2000m
16:00	1:07	1:43	2:18	2:55	3:34	4:53	6:11
16:10	1:08	1:44	2:20	2:57	3:36	4:56	6:15
16:20	1:09	1:45	2:22	2:59	3:39	4:59	6:19
16:30	1:10	1:46	2:23	3:01	3:41	5:03	6:23
16:40	1:10	1:48	2:25	3:03	3:43	5:06	6:27
16:50	1:11	1:49	2:27	3:05	3:46	5:09	6:31
17:00	1:12	1:50	2:28	3:07	3:48	5:12	6:35
17:10	1:13	1:51	2:30	3:09	3:51	5:16	6:39
17:20	1:14	1:53	2:31	3:11	3:53	5:19	6:43
17:30	1:14	1:54	2:33	3:13	3:55	5:22	6:47
17:40	1:15	1:55	2:35	3:15	3:58	5:25	6:51
17:50	1:16	1:56	2:36	3:17	4:00	5:28	6:55
18:00	1:17	1:57	2:38	3:19	4:03	5:32	7:00
18:10	1:18	1:59	2:39	3:21	4:05	5:35	7:04
18:20	1:19	2:00	2:41	3:23	4:08	5:38	7:08
18:30	1:19	2:01	2:43	3:25	4:10	5:41	7:12
18:40	1:20	2:02	2:44	3:27	4:12	5:44	7:16
18:50	1:21	2:03	2:46	3:29	4:15	5:48	7:20
19:00	1:22	2:05	2:47	3:31	4:17	5:51	7:24
19:10	1:23	2:06	2:49	3:33	4:20	5:54	7:28
19:20	1:23	2:07	2:51	3:35	4:22	5:57	7:32
19:30	1:24	2:08	2:52	3:37	4:24	6:01	7:36
19:40	1:25	2:09	2:54	3:39	4:27	6:04	7:40
19:50	1:26	2:11	2:56	3:41	4:29	6:07	7:44
20:00	1:27	2:12	2:57	3:43	4:32	6:10	7:48
20:10	1:27	2:13	2:59	3:45	4:34	6:13	7:52
20:20	1:28	2:14	3:00	3:47	4:36	6:17	7:56
20:30	1:29	2:15	3:02	3:49	4:39	6:20	8:00
20:40	1:30	2:17	3:04	3:51	4:41	6:23	8:04

5K-time	400m	600m	800m	1000m	1200m	1600m	2000m
20:50	1:31	2:18	3:05	3:53	4:44	6:26	8:08
21:00	1:31	2:19	3:07	3:55	4:46	6:30	8:12
21:10	1:32	2:20	3:08	3:57	4:49	6:33	8:16
21:20	1:33	2:21	3:10	3:59	4:51	6:36	8:20
21:30	1:34	2:23	3:12	4:01	4:53	6:39	8:24
21:40	1:35	2:24	3:13	4:04	4:56	6:42	8:28
21:50	1:35	2:25	3:15	4:06	4:58	6:46	8:32
22:00	1:36	2:26	3:16	4:08	5:01	6:49	8:36
22:10	1:37	2:28	3:18	4:10	5:03	6:52	8:40
22:20	1:38	2:29	3:20	4:12	5:05	6:55	8:44
22:30	1:39	2:30	3:21	4:14	5:08	6:59	8:48
22:40	1:39	2:31	3:23	4:16	5:10	7:02	8:52
22:50	1:40	2:32	3:24	4:18	5:13	7:05	8:56
23:00	1:41	2:34	3:26	4:20	5:15	7:08	9:00
23:10	1:42	2:35	3:28	4:22	5:18	7:11	9:04
23:20	1:43	2:36	3:29	4:24	5:20	7:15	9:08
23:30	1:43	2:37	3:31	4:26	5:22	7:18	9:12
23:40	1:44	2:38	3:33	4:28	5:25	7:21	9:16
23:50	1:45	2:40	3:34	4:30	5:27	7:24	9:20
24:00	1:46	2:41	3:36	4:32	5:30	7:27	9:24
24:10	1:47	2:42	3:37	4:34	5:32	7:31	9:28
24:20	1:47	2:43	3:39	4:36	5:34	7:34	9:32
24:30	1:48	2:44	3:41	4:38	5:37	7:37	9:36
24:40	1:49	2:46	3:42	4:40	5:39	7:40	9:40
24:50	1:50	2:47	3:44	4:42	5:42	7:44	9:44
25:00	1:51	2:48	3:45	4:44	5:44	7:47	9:48
25:10	1:51	2:49	3:47	4:46	5:46	7:50	9:52
25:20	1:52	2:50	3:49	4:48	5:49	7:53	9:57
25:30	1:53	2:52	3:50	4:50	5:51	7:56	10:01
25:40	1:54	2:53	3:52	4:52	5:54	8:00	10:05
25:50	1:55	2:54	3:53	4:54	5:56	8:03	10:09
26:00	1:56	2:55	3:55	4:56	5:59	8:06	10:13
26:10	1:56	2:56	3:57	4:58	6:01	8:09	10:17
26:20	1:57	2:58	3:58	5:00	6:03	8:13	10:21

5K-time	400m	600m	800m	1000m	1200m	1600m	2000m
26:30	1:58	2:59	4:00	5:02	6:06	8:16	10:25
26:40	1:59	3:00	4:01	5:04	6:08	8:19	10:29
26:50	2:00	3:01	4:03	5:06	6:11	8:22	10:33
27:00	2:00	3:03	4:05	5:08	6:13	8:25	10:37
27:10	2:01	3:04	4:06	5:10	6:15	8:29	10:41
27:20	2:02	3:05	4:08	5:12	6:18	8:32	10:45
27:30	2:03	3:06	4:10	5:14	6:20	8:35	10:49
27:40	2:04	3:07	4:11	5:16	6:23	8:38	10:53
27:50	2:04	3:09	4:13	5:18	6:25	8:41	10:57
28:00	2:05	3:10	4:14	5:20	6:28	8:45	11:01
28:10	2:06	3:11	4:16	5:22	6:30	8:48	11:05
28:20	2:07	3:12	4:18	5:24	6:32	8:51	11:09
28:30	2:08	3:13	4:19	5:26	6:35	8:54	11:13
28:40	2:08	3:15	4:21	5:28	6:37	8:58	11:17
28:50	2:09	3:16	4:22	5:30	6:40	9:01	11:21
29:00	2:10	3:17	4:24	5:32	6:42	9:04	11:25
29:10	2:11	3:18	4:26	5:34	6:44	9:07	11:29
29:20	2:12	3:19	4:27	5:36	6:47	9:10	11:33
29:30	2:12	3:21	4:29	5:38	6:49	9:14	11:37
29:40	2:13	3:22	4:30	5:40	6:52	9:17	11:41
29:50	2:14	3:23	4:32	5:42	6:54	9:20	11:45
30:00	2:15	3:24	4:34	5:44	6:57	9:23	11:49
30:10	2:16	3:25	4:35	5:46	6:59	9:27	11:53
30:20	2:16	3:27	4:37	5:48	7:01	9:30	11:57
30:30	2:17	3:28	4:38	5:50	7:04	9:33	12:01
30:40	2:18	3:29	4:40	5:52	7:06	9:36	12:05
30:50	2:19	3:30	4:42	5:54	7:09	9:39	12:09
31:00	2:20	3:31	4:43	5:56	7:11	9:43	12:13
31:10	2:20	3:33	4:45	5:58	7:13	9:46	12:17
31:20	2:21	3:34	4:47	6:00	7:16	9:49	12:21
31:30	2:22	3:35	4:48	6:02	7:18	9:52	12:25
31:40	2:23	3:36	4:50	6:04	7:21	9:56	12:29
31:50	2:24	3:38	4:51	6:06	7:23	9:59	12:33
32:00	2:24	3:39	4:53	6:08	7:25	10:02	12:37

5K-time	400m	600m	800m	1000m	1200m	1600m	2000m
32:10	2:25	3:40	4:55	6:10	7:28	10:05	12:41
32:20	2:26	3:41	4:56	6:12	7:30	10:08	12:45
32:30	2:27	3:42	4:58	6:14	7:33	10:12	12:50
32:40	2:28	3:44	4:59	6:16	7:35	10:15	12:54
32:50	2:29	3:45	5:01	6:18	7:38	10:18	12:58
33:00	2:29	3:46	5:03	6:20	7:40	10:21	13:02
33:10	2:30	3:47	5:04	6:22	7:42	10:24	13:06
33:20	2:31	3:48	5:06	6:24	7:45	10:28	13:10
33:30	2:32	3:50	5:07	6:26	7:47	10:31	13:14
33:40	2:33	3:51	5:09	6:28	7:50	10:34	13:18
33:50	2:33	3:52	5:11	6:30	7:52	10:37	13:22
34:00	2:34	3:53	5:12	6:32	7:54	10:41	13:26
34:10	2:35	3:54	5:14	6:34	7:57	10:44	13:30
34:20	2:36	3:56	5:16	6:36	7:59	10:47	13:34
34:30	2:37	3:57	5:17	6:38	8:02	10:50	13:38
34:40	2:37	3:58	5:19	6:40	8:04	10:53	13:42
34:50	2:38	3:59	5:20	6:42	8:07	10:57	13:46
35:00	2:39	4:00	5:22	6:44	8:09	11:00	13:50
35:10	2:40	4:02	5:24	6:46	8:11	11:03	13:54
35:20	2:41	4:03	5:25	6:48	8:14	11:06	13:58
35:30	2:41	4:04	5:27	6:50	8:16	11:10	14:02
35:40	2:42	4:05	5:28	6:52	8:19	11:13	14:06
35:50	2:43	4:06	5:30	6:54	8:21	11:16	14:10
36:00	2:44	4:08	5:32	6:57	8:23	11:19	14:14
36:10	2:45	4:09	5:33	6:59	8:26	11:22	14:18
36:20	2:45	4:10	5:35	7:01	8:28	11:26	14:22
36:30	2:46	4:11	5:36	7:03	8:31	11:29	14:26
36:40	2:47	4:13	5:38	7:05	8:33	11:32	14:30
36:50	2:48	4:14	5:40	7:07	8:35	11:35	14:34
37:00	2:49	4:15	5:41	7:09	8:38	11:39	14:38
37:10	2:49	4:16	5:43	7:11	8:40	11:42	14:42
37:20	2:50	4:17	5:44	7:13	8:43	11:45	14:46
37:30	2:51	4:19	5:46	7:15	8:45	11:48	14:50
37:40	2:52	4:20	5:48	7:17	8:48	11:51	14:54

5K-time	400m	600m	800m	1000m	1200m	1600m	2000m
37:50	2:53	4:21	5:49	7:19	8:50	11:55	14:58
38:00	2:53	4:22	5:51	7:21	8:52	11:58	15:02
38:10	2:54	4:23	5:53	7:23	8:55	12:01	15:06
38:20	2:55	4:25	5:54	7:25	8:57	12:04	15:10
38:30	2:56	4:26	5:56	7:27	9:00	12:07	15:14
38:40	2:57	4:27	5:57	7:29	9:02	12:11	15:18
38:50	2:57	4:28	5:59	7:31	9:04	12:14	15:22
39:00	2:58	4:29	6:01	7:33	9:07	12:17	15:26
39:10	2:59	4:31	6:02	7:35	9:09	12:20	15:30
39:20	3:00	4:32	6:04	7:37	9:12	12:24	15:34
39:30	3:01	4:33	6:05	7:39	9:14	12:27	15:38
39:40	3:02	4:34	6:07	7:41	9:17	12:30	15:43
39:50	3:02	4:35	6:09	7:43	9:19	12:33	15:47
40:00	3:03	4:37	6:10	7:45	9:21	12:36	15:51

TABLE 6.7

Key Run #2 Paces

(Improves lactate tolerance)

5K-time	(per mile)			(per kilometer)		
	Short Tempo	Mid Tempo	Long Tempo	Short Tempo	Mid Tempo	Long Tempo
16:00	5:26	5:41	5:56	3:22	3:32	3:41
16:10	5:29	5:44	5:59	3:24	3:34	3:43
16:20	5:32	5:47	6:02	3:26	3:36	3:45
16:30	5:36	5:51	6:06	3:28	3:38	3:47
16:40	5:39	5:54	6:09	3:30	3:40	3:49
16:50	5:42	5:57	6:12	3:32	3:42	3:51
17:00	5:45	6:00	6:15	3:34	3:44	3:53
17:10	5:49	6:04	6:19	3:36	3:46	3:55
17:20	5:52	6:07	6:22	3:38	3:48	3:57
17:30	5:55	6:10	6:25	3:40	3:50	3:59
17:40	5:58	6:13	6:28	3:42	3:52	4:01
17:50	6:01	6:16	6:31	3:44	3:54	4:03
18:00	6:05	6:20	6:35	3:46	3:56	4:05
18:10	6:08	6:23	6:38	3:48	3:58	4:07
18:20	6:11	6:26	6:41	3:50	4:00	4:09
18:30	6:14	6:29	6:44	3:52	4:02	4:11
18:40	6:17	6:32	6:47	3:54	4:04	4:13
18:50	6:21	6:36	6:51	3:56	4:06	4:15
19:00	6:24	6:39	6:54	3:58	4:08	4:17
19:10	6:27	6:42	6:57	4:00	4:10	4:19
19:20	6:30	6:45	7:00	4:02	4:12	4:21
19:30	6:34	6:49	7:04	4:04	4:14	4:23
19:40	6:37	6:52	7:07	4:06	4:16	4:25
19:50	6:40	6:55	7:10	4:08	4:18	4:27
20:00	6:43	6:58	7:13	4:10	4:20	4:29
20:10	6:46	7:01	7:16	4:12	4:22	4:31
20:20	6:50	7:05	7:20	4:14	4:24	4:33

5K-time	(per mile)			(per kilometer)		
	Short Tempo	Mid Tempo	Long Tempo	Short Tempo	Mid Tempo	Long Tempo
20:30	6:53	7:08	7:23	4:16	4:26	4:35
20:40	6:56	7:11	7:26	4:18	4:28	4:37
20:50	6:59	7:14	7:29	4:20	4:30	4:39
21:00	7:03	7:18	7:33	4:22	4:32	4:41
21:10	7:06	7:21	7:36	4:24	4:34	4:43
21:20	7:09	7:24	7:39	4:26	4:36	4:45
21:30	7:12	7:27	7:42	4:28	4:38	4:47
21:40	7:15	7:30	7:45	4:30	4:40	4:49
21:50	7:19	7:34	7:49	4:32	4:42	4:51
22:00	7:22	7:37	7:52	4:34	4:44	4:53
22:10	7:25	7:40	7:55	4:36	4:46	4:55
22:20	7:28	7:43	7:58	4:38	4:48	4:57
22:30	7:32	7:47	8:02	4:40	4:50	4:59
22:40	7:35	7:50	8:05	4:42	4:52	5:01
22:50	7:38	7:53	8:08	4:44	4:54	5:03
23:00	7:41	7:56	8:11	4:46	4:56	5:05
23:10	7:44	7:59	8:14	4:48	4:58	5:07
23:20	7:48	8:03	8:18	4:50	5:00	5:09
23:30	7:51	8:06	8:21	4:52	5:02	5:11
23:40	7:54	8:09	8:24	4:54	5:04	5:13
23:50	7:57	8:12	8:27	4:56	5:06	5:15
24:00	8:00	8:15	8:30	4:58	5:08	5:17
24:10	8:04	8:19	8:34	5:00	5:10	5:19
24:20	8:07	8:22	8:37	5:02	5:12	5:21
24:30	8:10	8:25	8:40	5:04	5:14	5:23
24:40	8:13	8:28	8:43	5:06	5:16	5:25
24:50	8:17	8:32	8:47	5:08	5:18	5:27
25:00	8:20	8:35	8:50	5:10	5:20	5:29
25:10	8:23	8:38	8:53	5:12	5:22	5:31
25:20	8:26	8:41	8:56	5:14	5:24	5:33
25:30	8:29	8:44	8:59	5:16	5:26	5:35
25:40	8:33	8:48	9:03	5:18	5:28	5:37

5K-time	(per mile)			(per kilometer)		
	Short Tempo	Mid Tempo	Long Tempo	Short Tempo	Mid Tempo	Long Tempo
25:50	8:36	8:51	9:06	5:20	5:30	5:39
26:00	8:39	8:54	9:09	5:22	5:32	5:41
26:10	8:42	8:57	9:12	5:24	5:34	5:43
26:20	8:46	9:01	9:16	5:26	5:36	5:45
26:30	8:49	9:04	9:19	5:28	5:38	5:47
26:40	8:52	9:07	9:22	5:30	5:40	5:49
26:50	8:55	9:10	9:25	5:32	5:42	5:51
27:00	8:58	9:13	9:28	5:34	5:44	5:53
27:10	9:02	9:17	9:32	5:36	5:46	5:55
27:20	9:05	9:20	9:35	5:38	5:48	5:57
27:30	9:08	9:23	9:38	5:40	5:50	5:59
27:40	9:11	9:26	9:41	5:42	5:52	6:01
27:50	9:14	9:29	9:44	5:44	5:54	6:03
28:00	9:18	9:33	9:48	5:46	5:56	6:05
28:10	9:21	9:36	9:51	5:48	5:58	6:07
28:20	9:24	9:39	9:54	5:50	6:00	6:09
28:30	9:27	9:42	9:57	5:52	6:02	6:11
28:40	9:31	9:46	10:01	5:54	6:04	6:13
28:50	9:34	9:49	10:04	5:56	6:06	6:15
29:00	9:37	9:52	10:07	5:58	6:08	6:17
29:10	9:40	9:55	10:10	6:00	6:10	6:19
29:20	9:43	9:58	10:13	6:02	6:12	6:21
29:30	9:47	10:02	10:17	6:04	6:14	6:23
29:40	9:50	10:05	10:20	6:06	6:16	6:25
29:50	9:53	10:08	10:23	6:08	6:18	6:27
30:00	9:56	10:11	10:26	6:10	6:20	6:29
30:10	10:00	10:15	10:30	6:12	6:22	6:31
30:20	10:03	10:18	10:33	6:14	6:24	6:33
30:30	10:06	10:21	10:36	6:16	6:26	6:35
30:40	10:09	10:24	10:39	6:18	6:28	6:37
30:50	10:12	10:27	10:42	6:20	6:30	6:39
31:00	10:16	10:31	10:46	6:22	6:32	6:41

5K-time	(per mile)			(per kilometer)		
	Short Tempo	Mid Tempo	Long Tempo	Short Tempo	Mid Tempo	Long Tempo
31:10	10:19	10:34	10:49	6:24	6:34	6:43
31:20	10:22	10:37	10:52	6:26	6:36	6:45
31:30	10:25	10:40	10:55	6:28	6:38	6:47
31:40	10:29	10:44	10:59	6:30	6:40	6:49
31:50	10:32	10:47	11:02	6:32	6:42	6:51
32:00	10:35	10:50	11:05	6:34	6:44	6:53
32:10	10:38	10:53	11:08	6:36	6:46	6:55
32:20	10:41	10:56	11:11	6:38	6:48	6:57
32:30	10:45	11:00	11:15	6:40	6:50	6:59
32:40	10:48	11:03	11:18	6:42	6:52	7:01
32:50	10:51	11:06	11:21	6:44	6:54	7:03
33:00	10:54	11:09	11:24	6:46	6:56	7:05
33:10	10:57	11:12	11:27	6:48	6:58	7:07
33:20	11:01	11:16	11:31	6:50	7:00	7:09
33:30	11:04	11:19	11:34	6:52	7:02	7:11
33:40	11:07	11:22	11:37	6:54	7:04	7:13
33:50	11:10	11:25	11:40	6:56	7:06	7:15
34:00	11:14	11:29	11:44	6:58	7:08	7:17
34:10	11:17	11:32	11:47	7:00	7:10	7:19
34:20	11:20	11:35	11:50	7:02	7:12	7:21
34:30	11:23	11:38	11:53	7:04	7:14	7:23
34:40	11:26	11:41	11:56	7:06	7:16	7:25
34:50	11:30	11:45	12:00	7:08	7:18	7:27
35:00	11:33	11:48	12:03	7:10	7:20	7:29
35:10	11:36	11:51	12:06	7:12	7:22	7:31
35:20	11:39	11:54	12:09	7:14	7:24	7:33
35:30	11:43	11:58	12:13	7:16	7:26	7:35
35:40	11:46	12:01	12:16	7:18	7:28	7:37
35:50	11:49	12:04	12:19	7:20	7:30	7:39
36:00	11:52	12:07	12:22	7:22	7:32	7:41
36:10	11:55	12:10	12:25	7:24	7:34	7:43
36:20	11:59	12:14	12:29	7:26	7:36	7:45

5K-time	(per mile)			(per kilometer)		
	Short Tempo	Mid Tempo	Long Tempo	Short Tempo	Mid Tempo	Long Tempo
36:30	12:02	12:17	12:32	7:28	7:38	7:47
36:40	12:05	12:20	12:35	7:30	7:40	7:49
36:50	12:08	12:23	12:38	7:32	7:42	7:51
37:00	12:12	12:27	12:42	7:34	7:44	7:53
37:10	12:15	12:30	12:45	7:36	7:46	7:55
37:20	12:18	12:33	12:48	7:38	7:48	7:57
37:30	12:21	12:36	12:51	7:40	7:50	7:59
37:40	12:24	12:39	12:54	7:42	7:52	8:01
37:50	12:28	12:43	12:58	7:44	7:54	8:03
38:00	12:31	12:46	13:01	7:46	7:56	8:05
38:10	12:34	12:49	13:04	7:48	7:58	8:07
38:20	12:37	12:52	13:07	7:50	8:00	8:09
38:30	12:40	12:55	13:10	7:52	8:02	8:11
38:40	12:44	12:59	13:14	7:54	8:04	8:13
38:50	12:47	13:02	13:17	7:56	8:06	8:15
39:00	12:50	13:05	13:20	7:58	8:08	8:17
39:10	12:53	13:08	13:23	8:00	8:10	8:19
39:20	12:57	13:12	13:27	8:02	8:12	8:21
39:30	13:00	13:15	13:30	8:04	8:14	8:23
39:40	13:03	13:18	13:33	8:06	8:16	8:25
39:50	13:06	13:21	13:36	8:08	8:18	8:27
40:00	13:09	13:24	13:39	8:10	8:20	8:29

TABLE 6.8

Key Run #3 Paces

(Skeletal and cardiac muscle adaptation)

5K-time	(per mile)		(per kilometer)	
	MP	**HMP**	**MP**	**HMP**
16:00	5:56	5:39	3:41	3:31
16:10	6:00	5:43	3:44	3:33
16:20	6:04	5:46	3:46	3:35
16:30	6:07	5:50	3:48	3:38
16:40	6:11	5:54	3:51	3:40
16:50	6:15	5:57	3:53	3:42
17:00	6:19	6:01	3:55	3:44
17:10	6:22	6:04	3:58	3:46
17:20	6:26	6:08	4:00	3:48
17:30	6:30	6:11	4:02	3:51
17:40	6:33	6:15	4:04	3:53
17:50	6:37	6:18	4:07	3:55
18:00	6:41	6:22	4:09	3:57
18:10	6:45	6:25	4:11	3:59
18:20	6:48	6:29	4:14	4:02
18:30	6:52	6:32	4:16	4:04
18:40	6:56	6:36	4:18	4:06
18:50	6:59	6:40	4:21	4:08
19:00	7:03	6:43	4:23	4:10
19:10	7:07	6:47	4:25	4:13
19:20	7:11	6:50	4:28	4:15
19:30	7:14	6:54	4:30	4:17
19:40	7:18	6:57	4:32	4:19
19:50	7:22	7:01	4:34	4:21
20:00	7:25	7:04	4:37	4:24
20:10	7:29	7:08	4:39	4:26
20:20	7:33	7:11	4:41	4:28

	(per mile)		(per kilometer)	
5K-time	MP	HMP	MP	HMP
20:30	7:37	7:15	4:44	4:30
20:40	7:40	7:18	4:46	4:32
20:50	7:44	7:22	4:48	4:35
21:00	7:48	7:25	4:51	4:37
21:10	7:51	7:29	4:53	4:39
21:20	7:55	7:33	4:55	4:41
21:30	7:59	7:36	4:58	4:43
21:40	8:02	7:40	5:00	4:46
21:50	8:06	7:43	5:02	4:48
22:00	8:10	7:47	5:04	4:50
22:10	8:14	7:50	5:07	4:52
22:20	8:17	7:54	5:09	4:54
22:30	8:21	7:57	5:11	4:57
22:40	8:25	8:01	5:14	4:59
22:50	8:28	8:04	5:16	5:01
23:00	8:32	8:08	5:18	5:03
23:10	8:36	8:11	5:21	5:05
23:20	8:40	8:15	5:23	5:08
23:30	8:43	8:19	5:25	5:10
23:40	8:47	8:22	5:27	5:12
23:50	8:51	8:26	5:30	5:14
24:00	8:54	8:29	5:32	5:16
24:10	8:58	8:33	5:34	5:19
24:20	9:02	8:36	5:37	5:32
24:30	9:06	8:40	5:39	5:23
24:40	9:09	8:43	5:41	5:25
24:50	9:13	8:47	5:44	5:27
25:00	9:17	8:50	5:46	5:30
25:10	9:20	8:54	5:48	5:32
25:20	9:24	8:57	5:51	5:34
25:30	9:28	9:01	5:53	5:36
25:40	9:32	9:04	5:55	5:38

	(per mile)		(per kilometer)	
5K-time	**MP**	**HMP**	**MP**	**HMP**
25:50	9:35	9:08	5:57	5:41
26:00	9:39	9:12	6:00	5:43
26:10	9:43	9:15	6:02	5:45
26:20	9:46	9:19	6:04	5:47
26:30	9:50	9:22	6:07	5:49
26:40	9:54	9:26	6:09	5:52
26:50	9:58	9:29	6:11	5:54
27:00	10:01	9:33	6:14	5:56
27:10	10:05	9:36	6:16	5:58
27:20	10:09	9:40	6:18	6:00
27:30	10:12	9:43	6:21	6:03
27:40	10:16	9:47	6:23	6:05
27:50	10:20	9:50	6:25	6:07
28:00	10:24	9:54	6:27	6:09
28:10	10:27	9:58	6:30	6:11
28:20	10:31	10:01	6:32	6:13
28:30	10:35	10:05	6:34	6:16
28:40	10:38	10:08	6:37	6:18
28:50	10:42	10:12	6:39	6:20
29:00	10:46	10:15	6:41	6:22
29:10	10:50	10:19	6:44	6:24
29:20	10:53	10:22	6:46	6:27
29:30	10:57	10:26	6:48	6:29
29:40	11:01	10:29	6:51	6:31
29:50	11:04	10:33	6:53	6:33
30:00	11:08	10:36	6:55	6:36
30:10	11:12	10:40	6:57	6:38
30:20	11:15	10:43	7:00	6:40
30:30	11:19	10:47	7:02	6:42
30:40	11:23	10:51	7:04	6:44
30:50	11:27	10:54	7:07	6:46
31:00	11:30	10:58	7:09	6:49

	(per mile)		(per kilometer)	
5K-time	MP	HMP	MP	HMP
31:10	11:34	11:01	7:11	6:51
31:20	11:38	11:05	7:14	6:53
31:30	11:41	11:08	7:16	6:55
31:40	11:45	11:12	7:18	6:57
31:50	11:49	11:15	7:20	7:00
32:00	11:53	11:19	7:23	7:02
32:10	11:56	11:22	7:25	7:04
32:20	12:00	11:26	7:27	7:06
32:30	12:04	11:29	7:30	7:08
32:40	12:07	11:33	7:32	7:11
32:50	12:11	11:37	7:34	7:13
33:00	12:15	11:40	7:37	7:15
33:10	12:19	11:44	7:39	7:17
33:20	12:22	11:47	7:41	7:19
33:30	12:26	11:51	7:44	7:22
33:40	12:30	11:54	7:46	7:24
33:50	12:33	11:58	7:48	7:26
34:00	12:37	12:01	7:50	7:28
34:10	12:41	12:05	7:53	7:30
34:20	12:45	12:08	7:55	7:33
34:30	12:48	12:12	7:57	7:35
34:40	12:52	12:15	8:00	7:37
34:50	12:56	12:19	8:02	7:39
35:00	12:59	12:22	8:04	7:41
35:10	13:03	12:26	8:07	7:44
35:20	13:07	12:30	8:09	7:46
35:30	13:11	12:33	8:11	7:48
35:40	13:14	12:37	8:14	7:50
35:50	13:18	12:40	8:16	7:52
36:00	13:22	12:44	8:18	7:55
36:10	13:25	12:47	8:20	7:57
36:20	13:29	12:51	8:23	7:59

5K-time	(per mile)		(per kilometer)	
	MP	HMP	MP	HMP
36:30	13:33	12:54	8:25	8:01
36:40	13:37	12:58	8:27	8:03
36:50	13:40	13:01	8:30	8:06
37:00	13:44	13:05	8:32	8:08
37:10	13:48	13:08	8:34	8:10
37:20	13:51	13:12	8:37	8:12
37:30	13:55	13:16	8:39	8:14
37:40	13:59	13:19	8:41	8:17
37:50	14:03	13:23	8:44	8:19
38:00	14:06	13:26	8:46	8:21
38:10	14:10	13:30	8:48	8:23
38:20	14:14	13:33	8:50	8:25
38:30	14:17	13:37	8:53	8:28
38:40	14:21	13:40	8:55	8:30
38:50	14:25	13:44	8:57	8:32
39:00	14:28	13:47	9:00	8:34
39:10	14:32	13:51	9:02	8:36
39:20	14:36	13:54	9:04	8:38
39:30	14:40	13:58	9:07	8:41
39:40	14:43	14:01	9:09	8:43
39:50	14:47	14:05	9:11	8:45
40:00	14:51	14:09	9:13	8:47

Training with Purpose: Q & A

Q. *When can I start my FIRST training?*

A. We recommend a training base of 15 miles (24 kilometers) per week for three months before beginning any of the FIRST programs; the base training for the Marathon Training Program should be closer to 25 miles (40 kilometers) per week. In addition to the requisite weekly miles, runners must be capable of long runs of 5 miles (8 kilometers) for the 5K Training Program, 6 miles (10 kilometers) for the 10K, 8 miles (13 kilometers) for the half-marathon and novice marathon, and 15 miles (24 kilometers) for the Marathon Training Program. If you are a beginning runner, see Chapter 4.

Q. *I have never done this type of training. How do I get started?*

A. During the base training, gradually become familiar with the track repeats and tempo runs. By introducing just one of the faster-paced workouts at a time, you can avoid too great a training overload at one time. During the base training and introduction to the FIRST training approach, these faster-paced workouts do not have to be run at a pace as fast as prescribed by FIRST for the training program. Use the three-month base training to gradually work up to your FIRST training efforts.

Q. *Can I use my goal race times to determine my training paces?*

A. It is important to determine training paces from actual race time performances, which represent your current fitness level. It needs to be emphasized that you should run the paces *based on your current fitness level* and not your goal race times. To do otherwise may increase your risk of incurring a running-related injury.

We have coached runners who insist on trying to run training paces consistent with their goal race times, rather than those determined from recent race performances. Recent race performances reflect your current fitness level. The problem that these runners encounter is in trying to maintain their ambitious training paces over several workouts. They may be able to meet the faster-than-their-current fitness level for Key Run #1 and, perhaps, even Key Run #2, but then fall apart in Key Run #3. In Chapter 11, we address running-related injuries due to overly ambitious training paces. The benefits of the FIRST program result from completing all the workouts week after week.

Q. *How important is it to stick to the prescribed paces?*

A. It is important to stay as close as possible to the prescribed paces—neither slower nor faster than the specified times. Again, while these runs may be challenging, they are not races. Running more slowly will not provide the stimulation necessary for adaptation; running faster will jeopardize your chances of successful completion of the next key workout. Furthermore, too fast a pace can lead to overtraining and possible injury.

Q. *When should I adjust the paces for faster workouts?*

A. Adjustment of training paces can be made after races that produce a new standard or after completing all three weekly workouts at the specified paces with the perceived exertion judged to be easy to moderate (that is, less than challenging). If either the race time indicates a faster training pace or if all three weekly workout times are easily achieved, then a faster pace should be attempted for the next week's workouts.

Q. *Why are there different recovery intervals?*

A. The workouts are designed to have a variety of distances and paces. Similarly, the recovery times for repeats are varied. The reason for training at different distances and intensities is that the body adapts when it is pressed to respond to an overload. Different types of overload elicit different physiological responses. The workouts are designed to stimulate the key physiological mechanisms needed for improved running performance. Recovery periods can increase or decrease the stress of the workouts. Varying the stressors—distance, pace, and recovery period—is a mechanism for producing changes in the workload and stimulating physiological adaptations.

Q. *How important are a warm-up and a cool-down?*

A. Your likelihood of achieving your target paces in your workouts will be enhanced with a proper warm-up. The ideal warm-up includes some dynamic stretching and a gradual intensity increase in your warm-up running. A cool-down will help to keep you from becoming stiff and sore later.

Q. *What if I don't have a track for Key Run #1?*

A. Runners who don't have a track for the repeats designated in Key Run #1 have several options. Find a flat section of road or path that has good footing and is safe for intense running, and measure and mark 400 meters. That will enable you to do most of the workouts. Another option is to use a GPS to measure the distance run. It can be programmed for distance or time.

Q. *Can I run only three times per week?*

A. We have conducted training studies that permitted runners to supplement our basic program with additional runs if they wished. What we found is that most runners chose not to do extra runs after the first few weeks because they found that they could perform the three Key Runs better with a day of recovery between workouts. There were no differences in the improvement of those who ran only three days per week, compared to those who did supplemental easy runs. For that reason, we designed the 3plus2 program to include the three quality runs and two cross-training workouts. An optional third cross-training workout is also permitted.

Running more than three times per week may be beneficial. Most running programs include running five to seven days per week. For reasons stated throughout this book, we find that much can be accomplished by running three times per week without the accompanying risks of injury.

The FIRST Training Programs don't restrict runners to only three runs per week, but any additional runs must not interfere with achieving the target paces of the three Key Runs. It is our experience that most runners do not run easily enough on "easy" run days. We have had runners report that they were successful by coupling one or two additional runs, but at relaxed and easy paces, with the three Key Runs prescribed by FIRST. As stated before, FIRST recommends coupling cross-training workouts with the three Key Runs so as to reduce the likelihood of injury and to provide more quality cardiorespiratory training.

Q. *Do I work out only three times a week?*

A. While we emphasize the importance of the three key running workouts to ensure the variety of stimulation needed for the primary physiological adaptations associated with a high level of fitness, the cross-training workouts—an essential part of the 3Plus2 Training Program—provide the additional training volume needed for development of aerobic endurance. The two components together offer the cardiorespiratory training that you would get in many popular training programs. In Chapter 7, the merits of cross-training are discussed and explained.

Q. *Isn't the FIRST 3Plus2 Training Program low on total training miles?*

A. There are many differences in individuals' abilities to tolerate training mileage. These differences are influenced by physiology, anatomy, biomechanics, and years of running experience. Typically, smaller, lighter, and younger runners are able to tolerate more miles. These runners become the elite performers who can run hard, run often, and run long. However, many runners—in particular, aging runners—find that they cannot tolerate high mileage weeks built on five to seven days of running. For them, reducing the number of days of running per week is appealing and effective. Runners with limited time for training, an injury, or who are just looking for a fresh approach to training may find that quality training can help them achieve faster performances while fitting their training into a balanced lifestyle. Because the FIRST program is lower on training miles than traditional running programs, it is attractive to those in the aforementioned categories. However, the FIRST 3Plus2 Training Program is *not* lower on training volume. A portion of the weekly total of aerobic training is achieved from aerobic modes of training other than running.

For a ballpark estimate of the number of equivalent miles you add to your training volume with cross-training, divide your total number of cross-training minutes by the average pace—number of minutes per mile or kilometer—you would normally maintain on a run for the number of run-equivalent miles or kilometers. For example, say you normally do a five-mile run at an 8:00/mile pace, but today you did 40 minutes of stationary biking at a comparable level of perceived exertion. Those 40 minutes of biking would equal five equivalent miles toward your weekly total training volume.

Q. *Will the low mileage program enable me to meet my running goals?*

A. Yes. Not only is this our belief, but it is also borne out by our own experiences and those of the runners we have trained and the many runners who have followed the FIRST Training Programs. By training with purpose, runners can achieve the high level of fitness necessary to improve their running performances (see the "Real Runner Report" at the end of this chapter). These three runs will require you to devote only three to five hours per week to running. The three sessions per week of high-quality running still provide you with the fitness benefits of high-intensity training and the stimulation, physiological and psychological, associated with hard efforts.

Q. *Will my fitness improve more with distance or intensity (speed)?*

A. Training volume and intensity are both critical factors in improving fitness. Runners often find it challenging to strike the right balance between volume and intensity. By running a lot of miles each week, it becomes difficult to run at a pace fast enough to stimulate the physiological adaptations needed to get faster and to build endurance. That's why FIRST incorporates three Key Run workouts with different distances and paces to develop a balance of endurance and speed.

Q. *Should I train the same way all year long?*

A. High school, collegiate, and elite runners have distinct running seasons. For high school and collegiate competitors, these seasons often consist of cross-country in the fall, indoor track in the winter, outdoor track in the spring, and base training in the summer. In the case of elite runners, their competitive schedules include the summer European track circuit and often a fall or spring road race, which, for the long-distance runners, means a major marathon. Thus, these competitors have specific championship races as goals, which determine their training schedules for their three or four annual peak performances. Conventional wisdom from exercise physiologists and elite coaches over the past 50 years suggests that training for these peak performances should be divided into distinct training periods, typically referred to as "periodization."

Q. *How can the age-group runner set up training phases compatible with racing goals?*

A. The year can be divided into cycles for one key race or up to four key races, one in each season. Race distances should allow ample time for recovery before the next cycle begins. FIRST does not recommend a four-race year that would include all marathons or even a combination of marathons and half-marathons.

Q. *What is an example of a year-round racing plan that incorporates different training phases?*

A. A training plan that includes a winter 5K, a spring 10K, a late-summer or early-fall half-marathon, and a fall marathon provides different types of training; these stimulate the physiological adaptations that determine running performance. Training programs must stimulate the body appropriately to produce workload adaptation. That is, for the 5K there must be more emphasis on intensity for shorter distances and for the marathon more emphasis on endurance.

If a marathon is in your yearlong plan, consider that a 16-week training plan, in addition to three to four weeks of recovery, covers five months. Developing specific training for shorter races and preparing for them specifically and properly requires several months. It is easy to see why developing a yearlong plan is important.

Q. *How can the FIRST three-quality-runs-per-week model be used for a year-round racing plan?*

A. The three basic workouts—track repeats, tempo, and long runs—can be used year-round as the basic training plan. You will notice that the training plans outlined in Chapter 6 are similar in structure, but the training distances are modified according to the race distance. Running the track repeats and tempo runs at a slightly faster pace becomes more important for the 5K and 10K preparation, and running the long runs at a slightly faster pace becomes more important for the half-marathon and marathon training.

Q. *How should I train when I am not following one of the FIRST Training Programs?*

A. We use the 3Plus2 Training Program year-round. In between the 12- or 16-week training programs, we still recommend doing an interval workout (Key Run #1), a tempo run (Key Run #2), and a long run (Key Run #3) to maintain fitness and to prepare for the next focused program. For variety, but to keep your training structured, you can do the following:

1. For Key Run #1, go to Tables 6.1–6.5 and choose "Track Repeats" workouts. You can make up a mixture of these.

2. For Key Run #2, do a 30- to 45-minute run with at least 15 to 35 minutes of running at a comfortably hard pace.

3. For Key Run #3, run between 10 and 15 miles if you are a half- or full marathoner or 6 to 8 miles if you are a 5K or 10K racer, so that you maintain your endurance and will be prepared to begin any of the training programs.

While you are doing similar workouts to what you will be doing in one of the FIRST Training Programs, the off-season training does not need to be as focused on pacing. You should rely more on perceived exertion. You can leave the watch at home. That is, you will give a good effort, but you won't have to worry about hitting the target paces that are an integral part of the FIRST Training Programs. The same advice can be applied to the cross-training. Choose different modes and enjoy the variety of workouts.

Q. *How does hill training fit into the 3Plus2 Training Program?*

A. The FIRST Training Program emphasizes the importance of maintaining the proper pace for all key workouts. We understand that the pace for a tempo run and a long run will be affected by hills and the topography of a course. More time will be lost on the uphills than gained on the downhills, but the two should even out roughly on an out-and-back or loop course. There is no easy rule for adjusting pace times for hills, since the steepness, total elevation gain, and length of the various inclines would have to be calculated.

Try to simulate racecourse terrain with your training course, if possible. If your planned race is on a hilly course, then train by using hills in longer runs as well as tempo runs. If you live in a flat area, you can treat bridges, overpasses, and parking decks as hills to incorporate hill training into your training. Hills certainly add stress to your training. That stress can make you a stronger runner. Learning to run hills economically takes practice. Obviously, it is tough to run your target paces over rolling, hilly courses. While your average pace over the distance of your run should be close to your target pace, you won't be running a constant pace, but you should be running at a constant effort. Your effort up and down hills should be the same. That means you will run more slowly than target pace up and faster than target pace down. You need to remain focused on the downhill sections of your run, which is where runners tend to relax. Staying focused on your effort for the duration and distance of your tempo and long runs will serve you well on race day.

Stress from hills not only taxes the cardiorespiratory system, it also stresses the muscles and connective tissue. Plantar fasciitis and Achilles tendonitis can develop from excessive hill running. Be sure to stretch the calves before and after hill running. I like running hills, but because of my tight calves I must limit the amount of time spent going up and down.

If you are headed to Boston in April, be sure to include hill training in your preparation. Be prepared to run several miles of uphill after miles of long, gradual downhill running that fatigues the quads. Most runners do not train for the downhill component of Boston.

Q. *Why is the longest marathon training run only 20 miles?*

A. There is no definitive study or theory for determining the optimal distance for the marathon long training run. I know runners who have run very good marathons with no run longer than 15 miles and runners who like to do at least one overdistance (that is, >26 miles) long run. Most marathon programs recommend long runs of 20 miles. Runs longer than 20 miles typically require additional recovery time, which then interferes with the following week's training. Where the threshold is located that stimulates adaptation and improvement, as opposed to the threshold that leads to prolonged fatigue, is a mystery. I am sure that it differs by individual, especially with the training pace of the individual. Consider that a 2:40 marathoner will complete a 20-mile training run in a little over two hours while a 5:00 marathoner will take four hours. Their recoveries from those efforts will be quite different.

We know that most marathoners stick to the 20-mile distance and are able to run excellent races with that preparation. FIRST recommends 20 miles as the longest training run because it is difficult to have a high-quality training run (meaning it is difficult to maintain a pace close to marathon pace) at a distance greater than 20 miles. So to run farther than 20 miles most likely will mean that you are running more slowly. Is it better to run 20 miles near marathon pace or to run farther at a slower pace? The FIRST Training Programs are based on pace, and our training philosophy is based on intensity. Intensity is the variable that contributes most to fitness. Thus, we prefer a long run that is faster than what most other programs recommend. That is the most distinctive characteristic of our training programs, along with running fewer days per week with potential additional runs replaced with cross-training.

Q. *Why does FIRST recommend five long training runs of 20 miles?*

A. Many runners ask, "Why so many?"; others, "Why so few?" There's nothing magical about five or any other number. We have had runners qualify for Boston with only one 20-mile run, using our Novice Marathon Program. There is no single training program that is ideal for everyone. However, in general, our experience in both running and coaching is that it's the long runs that best prepare you for the marathon. Too many long runs and your legs become fatigued; too few and you aren't trained to handle the race-day pace for the distance. We think five 20-mile runs over 15 weeks provide a good preparation.

Q. *Is it ever acceptable to do marathons back to back?*

A. Frequently, we get messages or calls from runners requesting help in how to train for a marathon four to eight weeks after a marathon they just finished. As noted above, we don't recommend running marathons so close together because you aren't going to get fitter with a few weeks of additional training, you are increasing your risk of injury, and you will not provide yourself with appropriate recovery time from the marathon you just completed. That said, there are times when it might be reasonable to try to get two marathons for the training for one. I worry about saying that because I don't want readers to take that as an endorsement for trying to piggyback marathons.

When is it OK to try a second marathon a short time after the first one? Say, you weren't feeling right, either before the race or a condition developed early in the race that caused you to run at training pace or more slowly. As a result, even though your performance was subpar, your recovery from the less taxing effort was more immediate, similar to a training run. The same could happen if race-day conditions were not conducive to an all-out effort. So, you decided to jog it because you were there and you like to collect medals, but you were smart enough not to try to defy physiology and attempt to run at your planned marathon pace; instead, you made it a prudent run around the city. In each of those cases it would be reasonable to consider another marathon in the next two months.

Depending on the level of stress the marathon caused and your assessment after a couple of days of any fatigue—general or specific—you could resume training. And if there is another marathon within the next four weeks, you could plan one more long run of 15 miles and then follow the last few weeks of the marathon training plan in Table 6.5. Yes, you would have two tapers for your training plan, but you have to figure that the 26.2-mile race, even if it was run at a slower than planned race pace, was probably more stressful than you are willing to admit, so it would be wise to be cautious about trying to squeeze any extra-hard work in for that next marathon.

If your second marathon is two months away, you could resume the marathon training plan starting at week 7 or 6 and follow it to the end.

This permission we are granting to run two marathons in close proximity does not apply to a hard effort that ended with a disappointing finish time. Even though there is an urge to redeem yourself immediately, your disappointment in almost every case becomes greater. Take a month to recover and then target your training for another marathon several months away.

Q. *Is it OK to use a race as my training run?*

A. This often-asked question stems from runners' enjoying participating in races. Most often, runners write and ask if it's OK to enter a local race and run it at the target training pace. If the race distance is shorter than their designated training run distance, they indicate that they will run some additional miles before or after the race. If the race is longer than their designated training run distance, they indicate that they will drop out once that distance has been completed. In theory, these strategies should not be a problem. In practice, intentions and reality do not match. Too often, runners write after the race that they were feeling good, the pace felt easy, and they were pulled along by the crowd and finished the race much faster than the target training pace or, in the case of the race being longer than their designated training distance, they were feeling good and decided not to drop out. Too often the targeted race and the preparation for it are undermined by using a race for training. Besides, why pay an entry fee for a training run?

Q. *I had a bad training run. What happened?*

A. Runners who are following the FIRST Training Program typically see their fitness improve and their training times get faster. After several weeks of improvement, they write us frantic after a poor training run—much slower than usual or, perhaps, they weren't able to complete it. It is common to have a bad run, as it is common to have a bad day. Why? We don't always know, but work, sleep, nutrition, cumulative fatigue, weather, and the various unknowns are among the factors. There is not just one Key Run in the 12- or 16-week training program; so, a bad run is not going to derail your preparation. Accept it as part of the training cycle and don't worry about it. It happens to everyone.

Q. *What should I do if I miss a workout? A whole week? Multiple weeks?*

A. Do not be concerned about a missed workout, nor should you try to squeeze it in later. Stay on schedule with the next workout and don't risk interfering with it. In particular, it's not a problem if you missed the workout because of your personal schedule. It becomes more complicated if you missed a workout because of injury. That's addressed in Chapter 11, "Running Injuries."

If you miss a week of training, that's typically not a problem, either. Over 16 weeks you aren't going to lose your fitness by missing a week. Again, continue with the schedule as if you had completed that missed week's training.

If you miss two or more weeks of training, you need to reconsider your target race and determine if your goal should be redirected to another race. It somewhat depends on when those two weeks were missed and why. If they were missed in the first four weeks of the training program, and you were reasonably fit when you began the training program, you can most likely continue with the training program without concern. If you missed the two weeks in the middle or near the completion of the training program, you will need to assess how much fitness was lost. More important is what you were doing during those two weeks. That is, if you were doing serious cross-training and staying fit, that's one thing. But if you were on a cruise, mostly inactive, and likely to have gained several pounds, that's a very different situation. I have heard from folks who reported both of the last two scenarios and my advice was quite different. The former was told to continue with the training program and the latter was told to pick another race as a goal.

Q. *Does FIRST recommend training with a heart rate monitor?*

A. FIRST does not use heart rate as a gauge of intensity for its key running workouts. We prefer using pace as a determinant of intensity. Heart rate fluctuations are caused by a range of variables and do not reflect running speed. A few of those variables, but not an exhaustive list, include body position, core temperature, hydration, emotions, time of day, lack of sleep, recovery status, nutritional status, and medications.

During a long run workout at a steady pace, your heart rate will increase initially and then level off as the oxygen requirement of the activity is met. However, prolonged exercise at a constant exercise intensity places an increasing load on the heart. Although the metabolic demands of the exercise do not increase, there is a progressive decrease in venous return of blood to the heart. So if venous return drops, there is less blood in the heart and stroke volume therefore drops. Your heart rate increases to compensate for the reduced stroke volume. The resulting decreased stroke volume and the accompanying increase in heart rate are referred to as "cardiovascular drift." This cardiac drift is generally due to decreased plasma volume caused by sweating. Thus, if you are maintaining a constant heart rate during that long run, you will gradually run more slowly throughout the run. Using heart rate to monitor effort on a long run won't prepare you to run a constant pace in your next race.

Q. *Can FIRST Key Runs be performed on a treadmill?*

A. Yes. Many runners have written us to report that they have done FIRST run workouts on a treadmill. Commonly, they do Key Runs #1 and #2 on the treadmill. Most report doing so because they need to run early in the morning or late at night and prefer not to run in the dark. Running in the dark increases the likelihood of an accidental injury. Runners from the North report performing their workouts on a treadmill when the ground is covered with snow and ice. Again, this is a wise choice to reduce the likelihood of an accidental injury. And the treadmill probably provides a better cardiorespiratory workout than a slower, cautious run on the slick outside surface. Runners from the South report doing summer workouts on the treadmill in an air-conditioned indoor space, rather than running more slowly in the extreme heat and humidity outside.

Our research shows that the oxygen and energy costs for running at a given pace are the same running on the treadmill as compared to running on the road. The treadmill does not need to be adjusted with elevation as long as the treadmill is calibrated accurately. That cannot be assumed. We find that belts on treadmills become loose and do not always travel at the speed that is displayed on the monitor. Runners often contact us for help in translating speed in miles-per-hour to minutes-per-mile. For that reason, we have provided a table in Appendix A of this book that provides those equivalencies.

Q. *How do I choose my race pace?*

A. For the half-marathon and marathon, your training program designates your HMP (half-marathon pace) and MP (marathon pace) from Table 6.8. That's your race pace. If during the 16-week training program you are able to do all three Key Runs without pushing yourself, you should use a faster 5K reference time for selecting your training targets and paces from Tables 6.6–6.8. That will result in a faster HMP and MP, which determine your target half-marathon and marathon target finish times. For the 5K Training Programs, your target race finish time is determined by your 5K reference time used for selecting training targets and paces. For the 10K target race finish time, refer to Table 3.1 and find the 10K time comparable to your 5K reference time.

Runners commonly write to ask why they should train at their most recent race time. They explain that they want to run faster at their next race. It's necessary to train at your current fitness level, which is best determined by your most recent race. That's the starting point for training. During the training, it is common to advance to a faster set of training paces, which indicates a faster race target finish time.

Q. *How does aging affect my ability to follow the FIRST Training Programs?*

A. Because training volume and intensity affect the three physiological factors that are the primary determinants of distance-running performance, the ability to sustain training levels is important. Aging affects training and recovery. Older runners often report that recovery from a hard workout takes longer than it once did and that they need a day of rest from running after each day of running. Reducing frequency and intensity of training impairs the optimal maintenance of physiological factors that determine performance potential. The FIRST training approach can help aging runners maintain intensity, even though they may reduce their running to three days per week. Finding another mode of training can complement the running to provide the training volume that contributes to a high level of fitness (see "Aging and Goal Setting," page 28).

Q. *What training pace adjustments need to be made at elevation?*

A. While the oxygen content of the atmosphere is at a constant percentage, 20.9% regardless of elevation, at higher elevations the atmospheric pressure decreases, reducing the partial pressure of oxygen, which makes less oxygen available for the runner. Endurance activities are hampered at higher elevations, beginning at around 3,000 feet. The extent of the performance reduction depends on the distance of the event and the extent to which the individual is acclimatized. The effects of elevation are greater on longer distances. At 5,000 feet elevation, you would expect a 3.5% reduction in performance in a 10K; at 7,500 feet elevation, you would expect a 6.3% reduction in performance in a 10K. See Chapter 10 ("Altitude Training and Racing") for altitude-adjustment tables.

||||||

REAL RUNNER REPORT

To All the Experts at FIRST,

I cannot thank you enough for your *Run Less Run Faster* book. Six months ago, I signed up for a marathon—my first in over 15 years. In my first marathon, my goal was simply to finish, and not to walk. I did that, and completed it in 4 hours and 10 minutes, which I felt great about! I knew then that I would run another marathon someday.

Someday ended up being 15 years and five children later! This time around, I wanted to qualify for the Boston Marathon and knew I would need some guidance as far as training goes. As a busy mom, I knew that I needed a training plan that took a little less time to execute, so when I heard about your 3plus2 method, I knew this was the plan for me. I ordered your book right away. When it arrived and I started browsing through it, I discovered that, based on my most recent half-marathon time, you believed I could run a marathon in 3:15. But I didn't believe it!! I thought I'd be pushing just to run a 3:40, the Boston qualifying standard for my age group. To run a 3:15 sounded like crazy talk!

But I decided to trust the experts and start training, following your Boston 3:15 plan. For the first few weeks, I was able to complete the tempo and long runs according to plan, but the speed interval times were a little out of reach. I felt a little frustrated and almost decided to back off my goal time a bit. But I kept deciding to try another week. In week seven, the magic finally happened! I had adapted to the speed work and finally hit the prescribed times! From there to the end, I was able to do it and felt confident heading into my race!

My race was on a downhill course, and I was tempted to take off way too fast. But I followed your advice and just ran a consistent pace—the 7:26 pace I had been training for. The first half of the race felt easy at this pace, and I had plenty of energy left to run strong to the finish. My second half was only 3 seconds slower than the first, and I finished in 3:15:14—EXACTLY what you said I could do!! I won my age division, was the fourth female overall, and am planning on running Boston in the spring!

Thanks for your expert training plan, and for believing in my potential. I never would have even attempted this feat if it wasn't for your knowledgeable resource and training plan. Thank you, thank you, thank you!!

Sincerely,

Taffy Micheli
Mother
Fort Bridger, Wyoming

7

Essential Cross-Training

The "2" of the 3Plus2 Training Program

The FIRST Training Program comprises three days of quality running and two days of cross-training. Although this approach has fewer days of running than many other running programs, the total volume of exercise is similar. While we suggest that runners actually run less, the FIRST program does not suggest that they exercise less.

We have received many messages from users of the FIRST program, describing how the cross-training component has provided welcome variety to their workouts. Many say they were surprised that adding cross-training made the running and the training week more enjoyable. In addition, they agreed that it enabled them to train harder than going for an easy run and that it helped them recover from the quality Key Runs.

From our FIRST Learning and Running Retreats, held on the Furman University campus, we have observed that most runners previously had not completed the cross-training workouts at the recommended intensity. Typically, each group of retreat runners finds that the cross-training workouts can also be fatiguing. They learn that the bike and rowing ergometer can be taxing when they are used in a focused workout. They find the same to be true of the pool.

Coauthor Scott Murr likes to say that he is a fit person who runs, rather than a runner who is fit. I suppose that, as physical educators, we are not as singularly focused as are many running coaches and authors. We are concerned about total fitness. Not only have we found that cross-training contributes to improved running, but it also enhances total fitness.

Total fitness is an important concept for runners who want to be running for a lifetime. Cross-training provides not only the cardiorespiratory endurance necessary for running success, but it also contributes to the muscular strength, muscular endurance, and flexibility needed to be a strong and enduring runner over many years. Cross-training also contributes to total fitness by improving body composition and helping runners develop the coordination and balance that reduce the likelihood of injury.

FIRST prefers non–weight-bearing activities—such as swimming, biking, and rowing—as cross-training activities to complement the three Key Runs. In this chapter we provide a cross-training program to accompany the three Key Runs. Combining these two training schedules provides a complete FIRST 3Plus2 Training Program.

Cross-Training: Q & A

Q. *How often should I cross-train?*

A. With the three key running workouts, include a minimum of two cross-training workouts per week. The number of cross-training sessions depends on the total training volume that is reasonable for your fitness level and available time for training, as well as the amount of running that you are doing. Some runners are able to tolerate and benefit from three or four cross-training workouts per week.

Q. *How long should cross-training sessions be?*

A. Rather than take a 30- to 45-minute easy run, you can cross-train at a higher intensity for the same duration. When cross-training, it is best to base workouts on time rather than distance. Just as with running, you can have short, intense cross-training workouts, made up of short high-intensity work intervals interspersed with rest bouts, or you can have workouts that mirror tempo workouts— a hard 20- to 25-minute effort—or you can have a workout that imitates the long run—a two- to three-hour moderate-intensity workout.

Q. *How do I measure the intensity of cross-training workouts?*

A. Many aerobic fitness machines have some built-in measure of work output or speed that you can use to judge your effort. While caloric displays on fitness equipment may not be an accurate estimate of your true caloric expenditure, they are usually consistent from day to day, which gives you a way to compare workouts. Perceived exertion is also a valid measure of exercise intensity. In other words, a 45-minute spin workout at a moderate cadence with little resistance may be an "easy" workout, while a 30-minute spin workout with a faster cadence and moderate resistance may be a "hard" workout.

For cross-training workouts, we ask runners to use perceived exertion for determining the intensity. Without knowing an individual's fitness level for a specific exercise mode or piece of equipment, it would be very difficult to recommend a specific workload—leg strength influences your workload on the bike and swimming technique greatly influences your lap times in the pool. Because heart rates vary for the same perceived effort from one mode to another, we do not use heart rates for determining exercise intensity.

Q. *Can I cross-train and run on the same day?*

A. Yes. Even though the 3plus2 program designates running and cross-training workouts on separate days, an individual seeking a high-volume training regimen can supplement the 3Plus2 Training Program with additional cross-training workouts on running workout days. Although most runners will not be eager to add extra training after the intense FIRST run workouts, cycling or swimming can be good cool-down recovery activities after a run. They are also ways of extending a run workout without extending the time of running-related muscular and connective tissue stresses. So that additional cross-training does not interfere with the Key Run, we recommend that those who want to cross-train and run on the same day complete their Key Run first.

Q. *What are the best cross-training activities for runners?*

A. It is important to choose activities that complement your running. The point is to give the running muscles a break. Activities such as swimming, rowing, and biking all offer good cardiovascular benefits without stressing your lower legs and running musculature. These are non–weight-bearing activities that help give the legs and running muscles a well-deserved break, promoting recovery.

Cross-training is an integral part of the FIRST training approach. It is important for you to avoid "all-or-nothing" thinking. New activities require time before you acquire a feel for the activity. Finally, as with running, it is important to learn the sense of proper pacing for the various modes of cross-training.

Q. *Can CrossFit or similar types of activities be used for cross-training?*

A. CrossFit and other similar approaches to exercise may be intense workouts, which can be beneficial for overall fitness. Some of the exercises used in fitness programs are very technique-dependent and if your form/technique is not good, the risk of injury is much greater.

Intense, short workouts may not be compatible with a runner's desire to get faster over a long distance. These intense workouts are often shorter than 20 minutes, with the focus primarily on the anaerobic component, rather than the aerobic component. Short and intense workouts may not be the best approach for helping a runner get faster for a 10K, a half-marathon, or marathon. The FIRST cross-training workouts are intended to further develop aerobic fitness.

CrossFit-type workouts should not be used as cross-training workouts in the FIRST 3Plus2 Training Program; however, these may contribute to a runner's muscular strength and endurance (see Chapter 14, "Strength Training for Runners") as long as they are not so muscularly intense that they have a detrimental impact on the next run workout.

Q. *Is spinning class acceptable for cross-training?*

A. Spin classes can be quite challenging. They can be good workouts every now and then. Most spin classes vary considerably in effort during the workout as a result of changes in resistance and spin rate. Spin classes are valuable because they can force you to work harder than you might otherwise.

Q. *Should I taper my cross-training before a race? How much?*

A. The goal for a runner is to arrive at the starting line of a race healthy, fit, rested, and ready to race. During the week leading up to the race, we recommend that runners reduce their training volume and skip the cross-training.

Q. *Does yoga count as cross-training?*

A. In general, yoga does not give runners the steady, rhythmic activity that provides the cardiorespiratory training needed for improving aerobic fitness. It definitely offers other benefits, such as flexibility, strength training, and core training; however, it is not a substitute for the aerobic cross-training recommended in our 3plus2 program.

Modes of Cross-Training

Cycling

Cycling is a non–weight-bearing and low-impact aerobic exercise that builds aerobic fitness while allowing recovery for the legs from the demands of running. It helps develop the quadriceps, which can balance the strengthening of the hamstrings and calves that results from running. Cycling can also increase hip and knee joint flexibility. Because there is no pounding with cycling, runners often recover quickly; therefore, cycling does not interfere too much with the demands of the Key Runs. Performing intervals on a bike can also help increase running cadence and contribute to improved running speed.

High-intensity bike intervals work the leg muscles even harder than uphill running, but without the impact of hard running. Cycling can be done outdoors, or indoors on a stationary trainer or bike.

For runners, cycling cadence is important. Most runners who cycle tend to "push a big gear" with a low cadence when cycling. Cycling is more beneficial when runners work on quick pedaling at a cadence of 80 to 100 pedal revolutions per minute.

If you choose to bike outdoors as a means of cross-training, you will find that cycling is much more expensive than running. Bikes cost more than running shoes. While running in the rain or cold may not be the most fun, most runners are able to run regardless of the weather. Cycling in the rain is no fun and can be quite risky. Cycling outside requires much more time than a comparable stationary bike workout. Although cyclists generally have fewer overuse injuries than runners, when a cyclist has a wreck, the injuries can be serious.

Indoor bike workouts may be a safer option than cycling outside. Indoor bike workouts can be social, fun, and do not require expensive equipment. With an indoor bike workout, runners are able to go at their own effort levels while still doing a group workout. Weather is not a factor.

There are a couple of drawbacks to indoor bike workouts. Not all stationary bikes have the necessary adjustments to provide a good fit. Because of the variety of indoor bikes, you may not be able to duplicate exact workloads and workouts. Many who cycle indoors often are distracted by their smartphones (e.g., texting, watching videos, etc.), which can reduce the intensity of the workout.

Swimming

Many runners who start to swim do so as a result of a running injury. Swimming is an excellent nonimpact way to improve overall fitness. Swimming increases upper-body strength and endurance while taking much of the stress off the legs. Swimming stretches the hamstrings and increases ankle flexibility, which may aid running performance. Swimming also allows the body to stay active, yet recover from a hard run.

Swimming requires much more technique than running. An unfit, skilled swimmer can typically outswim a fit runner lacking technique. Runners need to learn how to swim in a streamlined fashion. Once runners feel comfortable moving through the water, they can start building endurance. There is no doubt that swimming well requires time, commitment, and focused practice, but swimming is achievable for most runners.

While form and technique are important for running, they are much more so for swimming. Because most nonswimmers do not have good swim technique, they often get fatigued before they are able to get a good cardio workout from swimming; as a result, they do not swim regularly.

Swimming can be a great cross-training workout for runners, if they are patient and stick with it. For runners who want to incorporate swimming as part of their training, FIRST suggests that, just as with the run, you have a plan for the swim workout.

A reasonable goal for a runner would be to stay in the water for 30 minutes and move as much as possible. For example, swim one lap, rest 15 seconds, kick one lap using a kickboard, rest 15 seconds, and repeat this sequence for 30 minutes. You could look at this as an interval workout in the water.

Most runners hate kicking because they often feel as if they are working hard while making little progress down the pool; this is typically due to tight or inflexible ankles. Commit yourself to the kicking. You will get better and so will your lower leg and ankle flexibility; improved ankle flexibility can also impact running stride length.

If you do not give up on swimming, you will make quick gains. Just as with your running, set a goal for each workout. For example, the first short-range goal might be to swim 400 yards/meters nonstop, gradually increasing your goal to 1500 yards/meters.

Tips for Swimming (these are tips for runners who swim, rather than for competitive swimmers)

- Rather than swim with a fast arm turnover, strive to keep the strokes long and relaxed. Distance per stroke is more important than the number of strokes per minute. Concentrate on getting as much distance per stroke as you can. Count the number of strokes you take for one length of the pool; try to get your stroke count close to 20 (for a 25-yard pool).

- Develop good breathing technique; remember to exhale completely with your face in the water before rolling your head to the side to breathe. If you find that you are getting out of breath quickly, ask a swim instructor to offer some tips on your swim stroke.

- Since runners are accustomed to using their legs for propulsion, many runners who start swimming kick too hard. Swimming is primarily an upper-body activity since kicking only provides around 10% of the forward propulsion. Many runners kick hard because their kick is inefficient. Their kicking is inefficient because they have tight and inflexible ankles. Consequently, most runners do not like kick sets. However, kick sets not only help with aerobic fitness, but also help improve ankle and lower-leg flexibility.

Indoor Rowing

Indoor rowing is a good cross-training choice for runners. Rowing machines are widely available in fitness centers. Most runners are able to quickly learn the motion required.

Rowing is a total-body, non–weight-bearing exercise. It works both the upper and lower body, taking the major muscles through a wide range of motion, which promotes good flexibility.

Because it is an indoor activity, rowing can be done anytime. Finally, rowing is self-paced, so runners of all abilities can use it to develop their fitness.

Proper rowing technique is important to get the most out of the workout and to prevent injury. If you have not rowed using an ergometer, get instruction from a knowledgeable instructor on how to incorporate the legs, back, and arms. Proper technique can be learned easily. You can also find very good videos online showing the proper technique. Having an experienced rower watch and correct your technique will improve your efficiency and reduce injury risk.

Elliptical Fitness Machines and Stair Climbers

Stair climbing and elliptical fitness machines are increasingly popular in fitness clubs. Cross-training on an elliptical trainer allows you to duplicate running-like workouts in both time and intensity. Because they are weight-bearing modes that simulate running (without the pounding), this mode is not recommended for cross-training in the FIRST 3Plus2 Training Program. FIRST promotes cross-training in non–weight-bearing modes in an attempt to give the running muscles a chance to recover. Ellipticals are a viable substitute for running during recovery from certain types of injuries.

Stair climbers help build quadriceps strength, which helps with hill running. Because stair climbing is also a weight-bearing exercise, this mode is not recommended for cross-training in the FIRST Training Program.

Weight (Resistance) Training

Weight training or strength training is *not* considered cross-training in the FIRST Training Program. FIRST views cross-training, an aerobic workout without the pounding of the legs, as an activity designed to complement high-quality run training.

The Principle of Variation

The variation principle has several meanings. After quality run training, runners should cross-train to give their running muscles a chance to recover. The variation principle also refers to utilizing training cycles to vary the intensity and volume of training to help athletes achieve peak levels of fitness. The variation principle also means that athletes should change their exercises or activities periodically so that they do not overstress a particular part of the body. Changing activities also helps runners maintain their interest in running. The FIRST Training Program includes variation in paces. Each workout in the FIRST Training Program is completed at different paces.

It may appear that the specificity principle and the variation principle are incompatible. The specificity principle states that training must be specific to the desired adaptation and the variation principle seemingly asserts the opposite: Train by using a variety of activities. The incompatibility is resolved by the degree to which each principle is followed. More specific training is better to the extent that it can be tolerated, but it can become exceedingly boring and risky. Thus, some variety that involves the same muscle groups is a useful change.

FIRST Cross-Training Workouts

Below are descriptions of cross-training workouts that will enhance your running. As we have stressed throughout this book, substituting different modes of aerobic training for running workouts can have multiple benefits—reduced likelihood of an overuse injury, increased recovery time for running muscles, variety in training, and even increased training intensity. Suggested cross-training workouts appear in Tables 7.1–7.4.

We provide a progressive cross-training program that accompanies the 5K and 10K Training Programs and one that accompanies the Half-Marathon and Marathon Training Programs. The cross-training programs provide two bike workouts, a rowing workout, and a swimming workout in conjunction with the 16-week run training programs.

Runners should select two cross-training workouts for the corresponding week of their run training. These workouts complement the three key running workouts and are an integral part of the FIRST Training Program.

You can repeat a workout twice or you can choose to perform a workout of a different mode. FIRST recommends that you choose different workouts and different modes for variety. That helps to keep the workouts fresh.

Most runners use cycling as their primary choice for cross-training. Tables 7.1 and 7.3 include two cycling cross-training workouts for each week for the 5K and 10K Training Programs and the Half-Marathon and Marathon Training Programs, respectively. The cross-training workouts for the longer race distances are lengthier.

Tables 7.2 and 7.4 include rowing and swimming workouts for each of the training weeks for the 5K and 10K and Half-Marathon and Marathon Training Programs, respectively.

Because there is no comparable measure of intensity among different types of equipment, we suggest that runners use perceived effort as a measure of cross-training effort level or intensity. The effort levels for the cross-training workouts are described in terms related to your Key Run workout efforts.

For example, a cross-training workout labeled as "tempo" would be similar to the perceived effort of a Key Run #2 tempo run. A "hard" effort would be similar to the perceived effort of a Key Run #1 track repeat. An "easy" workout is comparable in effort to a warm-up, cool-down, or recovery interval.

TABLE 7.1

Cycling Workouts for 5K and 10K Training

Easy = Effort similar to warm-up and cool-down; Tempo = Effort similar to Key Run #2; Hard = Effort similar to Key Run #1.

Reminder: Cycling translates well to running when runners maintain a quick cadence of 80 to 100 rpm (revolutions per minute) during easy/relaxed, tempo, and hard efforts.

WEEK	CYCLING WORKOUT #1	CYCLING WORKOUT #2
12	10 min Easy 8 min Tempo 7 min Easy	10 min Easy 10 min Tempo 5 min Easy
11	10 min Easy 2 x (2 min Hard, 2 min Easy) 5 min Easy	10 min Easy 14 min Tempo 6 min Easy
10	20 min Tempo, gradually increasing the effort as the workout progresses from 5 min to 20 min	5 min Easy 15 min Tempo 5 min Easy
9	10 min Easy 2 x (1 min Hard, 3 min Easy) 5 min Easy	10 min Easy 5 min Tempo 5 min Easy 5 min Hard 5 min Easy
8	8 min Easy 15 min Tempo 7 min Easy	10 min Easy 5 x (1 min Hard, 4 min Easy) 5 min Easy

WEEK	CYCLING WORKOUT #1	CYCLING WORKOUT #2
7	10 min Easy 10 min Tempo 5 min Easy 10 min Tempo 5 min Easy	10 min Easy 8 min Hard 5 min Easy 7 min Hard 5 min Easy
6	10 min Easy 2 x (10 min Tempo-run ½ mile at MP) 5 min Easy	25 min Tempo, gradually increasing the effort as the workout progresses from 5 min to 20 min
5	10 min Easy 6 x (1 min Hard, 4 min Easy) 5 min Easy	10 min Easy 10 min Tempo 10 min Easy 5 min Hard 5 min Easy
4	10 min Easy 30 min Tempo, followed immediately by 10 min of Easy running	30 min Easy
3	10 min Easy 30 min Tempo 5 min Easy	10 min Easy 2 x (2 min Tempo, 2 min Easy) 5 min Easy
2	10 min Easy 20 min Tempo 10 min Easy	30 min Easy
1	Race Week During the week leading up to your race, you may skip the cross-training. The primary goal is to get to the starting line rested and feeling ready to run your best.	

TABLE 7.2

Rowing and Swimming Workouts for 5K and 10K Training

Easy = Effort similar to warm-up and cool-down; Tempo = Effort similar to Key Run #2; Hard = Effort similar to Key Run #1.

WEEK	ROWING WORKOUTS	SWIMMING WORKOUTS
12	8 min Easy 3 min Tempo 3 min Easy	20 x (kick 1 length, rest 30 sec) using a kickboard
11	7 min Easy 4 min Tempo 5 min Easy	12 x (swim 1 length, rest 15 sec, kick 1 length, rest 20 sec)
10	5 min Easy 4 x (1 min Hard, 1 min Easy) 4 min Easy	20 x (kick 1 length, rest 20 sec) using a kickboard
9	5 min Easy 2 x (3 min Tempo, 1 min Easy) 5 min Easy	Swim (any stroke) and kick for 20 nonstop min in any combination
8	5 min Easy 12 min Tempo 3 min Easy	5 x (kick 2 lengths, rest 15 sec, swim 2 lengths, rest 30 sec)

WEEK	ROWING WORKOUTS	SWIMMING WORKOUTS
7	10 min Easy 15 min Tempo 5 min Easy	3 x the following set with 1 min rest after set (swim 1 length Fast, 1 length Easy 2 lengths Fast, 2 lengths Easy 3 lengths Fast, 3 lengths Easy 2 lengths Fast, 2 lengths Easy 1 length Fast, 1 length Easy)
6	5 min Easy 1 min Hard, 1 min Easy 2 min Hard, 1 min Easy 3 min Hard, 1 min Easy 4 min Hard, 1 min Easy 3 min Hard, 1 min Easy 2 min Hard, 1 min Easy 1 min Hard, 3 min Easy	5 x (swim 8 lengths immediately followed by kicking 2 lengths) rest 1 min between sets
5	5 min Easy 10 min Tempo 5 min Easy 10 min Tempo 5 min Easy	25 min of nonstop moving in the water, using a combination of swimming and kicking
4	5 min Easy 4 x (3 min Hard, 2 min Easy) 5 min Easy	10 x (swim 2 lengths, rest 15 sec) Kick 4 lengths 10 x (swim 2 lengths, rest 15 sec)

WEEK	ROWING WORKOUTS	SWIMMING WORKOUTS
3	5 min Easy 1 x (4 min Hard, 1 min Easy) 4 x (1 min Hard, 1 min Easy) 2 x (3 min Hard, 1 min Easy) 4 x (1 min Hard, 1 min Easy) 4 min Easy	Swim 4 lengths Easy 3 x (swim 2 lengths Easy, swim 2 lengths Fast, rest 30 sec) 6 x (swim 1 length Easy, swim 1 length Fast, rest 15 sec)
2	5 min Easy 20 min Tempo 5 min Easy	Kick 4 lengths Swim 20 min Kick 4 lengths
1	Race Week During the week leading up to your race, you may skip the cross-training. The primary goal is to get to the starting line rested and feeling ready to run your best.	

TABLE 7.3

Cycling Workouts for Half-Marathon and Marathon Training

Easy = Effort similar to warm-up and cool-down; Tempo = Effort similar to Key Run #2;
Hard = Effort similar to Key Run #1.

Reminder: Cycling translates well to running when runners maintain a quick cadence of
80 to 100 rpm (revolutions per minute) during easy/relaxed, tempo, and hard efforts.

WEEK	CYCLING WORKOUT #1	CYCLING WORKOUT #2
16	10 min Easy 10 min Tempo 10 min Easy	10 min Easy 3 x (2 min Hard, 2 min Easy) 10 min Easy
15	10 min Easy 10 min Tempo 2 min Easy 3 min Hard 5 min Easy	10 min Easy 2 x (1 min Hard, 3 min Easy) 5 min Easy
14	10 min Easy 20 min Tempo 10 min Easy	10 min Easy 5 x (1 min Hard, 1 min Easy) 10 min Easy
13	10 min Easy 8 min Hard 2 min Easy 8 min Hard 10 min Easy	30 min Easy

WEEK	CYCLING WORKOUT #1	CYCLING WORKOUT #2
12	10 min Easy 30 min Tempo	5 min Easy 3 x (5 min Tempo, 1 min Easy) 5 min Easy
11	10 min Easy 15 min Tempo 5 min Easy 10 min Tempo 5 min Easy	35 min Easy
10	10 min Easy 20 min Tempo 5 min Easy 10 min Tempo 5 min Easy	5 min Easy 1 min Hard, 1 min Easy 2 min Hard, 1 min Easy 3 min Hard, 1 min Easy 4 min Hard, 1 min Easy 3 min Hard, 1 min Easy 2 min Hard, 1 min Easy 1 min Hard, 3 min Easy
9	10 min Easy 6 x (2 min Hard, 3 min Easy) 10 min Easy	20 min Easy 10 min Tempo 10 min Easy
8	10 min Easy 1 min Hard, 1 min Easy 2 min Hard, 1 min Easy 3 min Hard, 1 min Easy 3 min Hard, 1 min Easy 2 min Hard, 1 min Easy 1 min Hard, 3 min Easy	20 min Easy 5 min Tempo 15 min Easy

WEEK	CYCLING WORKOUT #1	CYCLING WORKOUT #2
7	10 min Easy 15 min Tempo 5 min Easy 10 min Tempo 5 min Easy	10 min Easy 5 x (2 min Hard, 3 min Easy) 10 min Easy
6	8 min Easy 7 x (1 min Hard, 2 min Easy) 8 min Easy	15 min Easy 10 min Tempo 15 min Easy
5	5 min Easy 15 min Tempo 5 min Easy 10 min Tempo 10 min Easy	10 min Easy 8 x (1 min Hard, 4 min Easy) 5 min Easy
4	10 min Easy 20 min Tempo 10 min Easy	20 min Easy 5 min Tempo 15 min Easy
3	10 min Easy 30 min Tempo 5 min Easy	10 min Easy 3 x (2 min Hard, 3 min Easy) 10 min Easy
2	15 min Easy 15 min Tempo 5 min Hard 10 min Easy	10 min Easy 3 x (2 min Tempo, 2 min Easy) 10 min Easy
1	Race Week During the week leading up to your race, you may skip the cross-training. The primary goal is to get to the starting line, rested and feeling ready to run your best.	

TABLE 7.4

Rowing and Swimming Workouts for Half-Marathon and Marathon Training

Easy = Effort similar to warm-up and cool-down; Tempo = Effort similar to Key Run #2; Hard = Effort similar to Key Run #1.

WEEK	ROWING WORKOUTS	SWIMMING WORKOUTS
16	8 min Easy 10 min Tempo 5 min Easy	20 x (kick 1 length, rest 30 sec) using a kickboard
15	7 min Easy 1 min Hard, 1 min Easy 2 min Hard, 1 min Easy 2 min Hard, 1 min Easy 1 min Hard, 4 min Easy	12 x (swim 1 length, rest 15 sec, kick one length, rest 20 sec)
14	10 min Easy 10 min Tempo 5 min Easy	20 x (kick 1 length, rest 20 sec) using a kickboard
13	10 min Easy 5 min Hard 5 min Easy	Swim (any stroke) and kick for 20 nonstop min in any combination
12	10 min Easy 5 min Tempo 5 min Hard 5 min Easy	5 x (kick 2 lengths, rest 15 sec, swim 2 lengths, rest 30 sec)

WEEK	ROWING WORKOUTS	SWIMMING WORKOUTS
11	10 min Easy 5 x (1 min Hard, 1 min Easy) 5 min Easy	5 x (swim 8 lengths immediately followed by kicking 2 lengths) rest 1 min between sets
10	5 min Easy 1 min Hard, 1 min Easy 2 min Hard, 1 min Easy 3 min Hard, 1 min Easy 4 min Hard, 1 min Easy 3 min Hard, 1 min Easy 2 min Hard, 1 min Easy 1 min Hard, 3 min Easy	3 x (swim 1 length Hard, 1 length Easy, 2 lengths Hard, 2 lengths Easy, 3 lengths Hard, 3 lengths Easy, 2 lengths Hard, 2 lengths Easy, 1 length Hard, 1 length Easy) rest 1 min between sets
9	5 min Easy 10 min Tempo 3 min Easy 10 min Tempo 5 min Easy	25 min of nonstop moving in the water, using a combination of swimming and kicking
8	5 min Easy 5 x (3 min Hard, 1 min Easy cycling) 5 min Easy	10 x (swim 2 lengths, rest 15 sec) Kick 4 lengths 10 x (swim 2 lengths, rest 15 sec)
7	5 min Easy 10 x (1 min Hard, 1 min Easy) 4 min Easy	Swim 4 lengths Easy 3 x (swim 2 lengths Easy, 2 lengths Fast, rest 30 sec) 6 x (swim 1 length Easy, 1 length Fast, rest 15 sec)

WEEK	ROWING WORKOUTS	SWIMMING WORKOUTS
6	5 min Easy 6 x (3 min Hard, 1 min Easy) 5 min Easy	Kick 4 lengths Swim 20 min Kick 4 lengths
5	5 min Easy 15 min Tempo 5 min Easy	20 x (kick 1 length, 　　rest 15 sec) using a 　　kickboard Swim 20 lengths nonstop
4	5 min Easy 5 min Tempo 5 min Easy 5 min Tempo 5 min Easy	Kick 4 lengths Swim 20 min Kick 4 lengths
3	5 min Easy 1 x (4 min Hard, 1 min Easy) 4 x (1 min Hard, 1 min Easy) 3 x (2 min Hard, 1 min Easy) 2 x (3 min Hard, 1 min Easy) 4 x (1 min Hard, 1 min Easy) 5 min Easy	3 x (swim 1 length Hard, 1 length 　　Easy, 2 lengths Hard, 　　2 lengths Easy, 3 lengths 　　Hard, 3 lengths Easy, 　　2 lengths Hard, 2 lengths 　　Easy, 1 length Hard, 1 length 　　Easy) rest 1 min between sets
2	10 min Easy 10 min Tempo 5 min Easy	10 x (kick 1 length the pool, 　　rest 15 sec) using a 　　kickboard Swim 20 lengths nonstop
1	Race Week During the week leading up to your race, you may skip the cross-training. The primary goal is to get to the starting line rested and feeling ready to run your best.	

REAL RUNNER REPORT

Dr. Pierce & Dr. Murr,

I'm a big fan of your book *Run Less Run Faster*, and I tell all my running friends how much it's benefited me! I picked consistent running back up in my life in 2012 (I had been on and off since 2007) and have run at least two half-marathons a year since 2013. I initially just stuck to a generic half-marathon training plan I found online, usually with four runs a week and no cross-training.

However, I got into triathlons and started taking a spin class twice a week, so I dropped down to three weekly runs with two days of spinning and saw no decrease in performance/fitness. This was before I heard about *Run Less Run Faster*, so when I did read about your book in *Runner's World* a couple years ago, I was excited to get it because my personal experience had already affirmed your basic premise. I devoured the book and learned more about speed work (which I had not consistently incorporated into my training . . . never on a track) and training with purpose to improve targeted running metrics.

The three subsequent halfs that I ran (all using your 16-week training plan) all set new PRs for me! I had been at 1:28:21 for a few years, then dropped to 1:28:09, then 1:27:12 seven months later, then 1:24:29 five months after that, at the age of 35!

Like I said above, I tell all my running friends about your book and plan, and I have the results to back it up!

> Thanks!
> Adam Sandwick
> Accountant
> Enid, Oklahoma

8

Rest and Recovery

A basic principle of training is overload. Overload is a planned, systematic, and progressive increase in training stress in order to improve fitness and/or performance. In other words, train hard and become fatigued, then rest and recover while the body accommodates the need to adapt to an increased workload. Repeating this training cycle of overload, fatigue, recovery, and adaptation leads to a fitter and faster runner. However, the fitness adaptation occurs during the recovery phase of this training cycle and there is a limit to one's capacity to endure and adapt. The progressive overload must be done gradually.

An overload for runners can mean running farther, more often, or faster. It is important that these stressors be gradually increased separately and care must be taken not to increase multiple stressors simultaneously. In other words, overload only one variable at a time.

Other nontraining stressors can add to your overload. These nontraining stressors include elevation, colds and allergies, poor dietary habits, environmental extremes, travel, stressful work situations, and stressful personal relationships. Pay attention to elevated outside stressors and recognize when it might not be a good time to increase your training load.

Most runners tend to think that more training (the overload aspect of the training cycle) will make them faster. To a certain extent that is true. However, crossing your threshold of tolerance for increased stress will result in fatigue that exceeds the body's ability for adaptation. Highly competitive, goal-oriented runners are vulnerable to the lure of dedicating themselves to incessant training with expectations of significant performance improvements. Those dedicated efforts can prove to be unproductive.

The key to getting faster is to combine the appropriate amount of quality training with quality rest and recovery. Increasing the overload at a rate that exceeds the body's ability to adapt causes staleness and even exhaustion. This condition of overtraining results in an impaired ability to train and perform. If any component of a training program—frequency, intensity, or duration—is increased too rapidly or if the program does not provide adequate recovery from the increased demands, a runner will suffer from the inability to adapt. This inability will lead to a decline in performance. Recovery and rest are essential components of a training program.

Runners are told to listen to their bodies. Recognizing the signs and symptoms of overtraining early, and intervening in the cycle with increased rest before fatigue becomes chronic, are both important. Those symptoms of overtraining include mood disturbances, irritability, sleep disturbances, increased susceptibility to colds, appetite changes, and a struggle to maintain standard training performances. Rest and recovery are essential for counteracting the fatigue created from the training overload necessary for adaptation.

What Aids Recovery?

In a recent book, *Good to Go*, Christie Aschwanden tackles the topic of how the human body can best recover and adapt to sports and fitness training. She examines the many trendy methods and products for enhancing recovery from training. Because both professional and amateur athletes are always looking for a competitive edge, entrepreneurs are eager to tout the latest product or service that will lead to a better performance. Aschwanden describes her experimentation with many of these services and products, and examines research studies for validation of their efficacy.

Interestingly, her conclusions about recovery, after a near-exhaustive examination of the multibillion-dollar recovery industry, are much the same as what we offered as advice in the previous edition of this book: "Listen to your body and learn to recognize the signs and symptoms of overtraining." Overcome the urge to do more when your body is desperate for rest.

Are there products and services that can aid your recovery? For the most part, you will have to determine that through experimentation. Whether it is a special sports drink, a massage, an ice bath, cupping, a foam roller, a sleep tracker, a special diet, or meditation, you can find successful athletes who attest to the effectiveness of each method or product. The science of recovery offers scant evidence for most of these products or strategies. Adequate sleep and rest from training are the exceptions to these other unproven recovery aids. Sleep and rest are universally mentioned as essential for peak performances.

What about runners who haven't missed a day for years (known as "streakers"), or those who run a marathon every week? Yes, there are runners who use the words *rest* and *recovery* with disdain. Many runners have the idea that runners are "tough" and think that rest and recovery are signs of weakness. However, rest and recovery are training tools that should be included in any training program. Streakers are typically more concerned with their streaks than they are with their performance potential. Runners who are overloading without recovery are vulnerable to injury and illness. Besides compromising their immune systems and increasing their susceptibility to a running-related malady, streakers most likely will not be able to perform to their full potential.

Rest and Recovery: Q & A

Q. *When is it important to rest and recover?*

A. Once you have completed a key workout or a race, it is important to recover from that training effort. The FIRST training approach balances quality runs with quality rest and recovery. The day following a Key Run workout is intended to be a rest day for the weight-bearing running muscles. The point is to give the legs a chance to recover so that the next key run can be a quality and productive run.

Q. *What influences the rate of recovery?*

A. The rate of recovery is influenced by many factors, including age, fitness level, exercise background and experience, life stressors, health level, diet, and sleep. Finding the appropriate balance of overload and recovery is essential for improvement. We have developed training schedules with prescribed distances and paces to provide the overload needed to stimulate adaptation. By gradually increasing the pace or distance, the body will continue to adapt and you will become fitter.

Q. *How should a recovery be structured during a training period?*

A. Recovery during training can refer to recovery in a workout or between workouts. With the FIRST training approach, runners perform three Key Runs in any order throughout the week; however, they need to allow for recovery between the Key Runs. We recommend that runners cross-train on other days of the week. The idea is to give the primary running muscles an opportunity to recover so that an optimal training load can be applied at the next scheduled run workout. Combined with sound nutrition, non-running days allow the opportunity for muscle glycogen to be replenished.

Rest prior to a stressful run (a FIRST Key Run or a race) allows the runner the best opportunity to complete the run at the necessary intensity. We have found that most runners who try to maintain their five-days-per-week running routine are unable to complete the Key Run workouts at the prescribed intensities. A non-running day prior to the Key Run serves as a mini-taper.

Q. *What can be done to enhance recovery?*

A. We mentioned in Chapter 6 that a cool-down after the Key Runs will aid in preventing soreness and stiffness. We also recommend post-workout static stretching as an important component of recovery (see Chapter 15, "Flexibility and Form"). Doing yoga or Pilates is reported by many runners to be a key to recovery from run workouts. Massage helps my recovery and when I am without access to a good massage or physical therapist, a foam roller has provided me with remarkable relief from muscular tightness.

Q. *How should recovery be structured for a pre-race event?*

A. If you are training to race, it is important to allow your body to recover from the stresses of prolonged training periods, assuming that your goal is to run your best. You cannot maintain your normal training schedule and then go straight into a race and expect to run a PR.

Pre-race rest does not necessarily mean one or two days without running or exercise before race day. A pre-race rest period must be significant and must be structured. In a structured training schedule, training builds up gradually (with built-in recovery periods) until some specified period before the target race when the training load usually peaks. Then a taper begins with a reduced training load, generally two weeks before a marathon and one week before a 5K or 10K. This taper allows the body to thoroughly recover. Then athletes are fully prepared to race and can reasonably expect to perform at or near their best. All FIRST Training Programs include a taper prior to a race.

Q. *How should post-race recovery be structured?*

A. Once you have completed a race, it is important to recover from that stress. Improvement occurs during the recovery phase and not the workout itself. The rate of recovery is influenced by many factors. One key recovery factor is post-run hydration/nutrition (see Chapter 12 on nutrition for post-exercise/race recommendations).

Because of the stress of a race, you cannot expect to return to pre-race levels of training immediately. The body needs time to recover. An immediate return to high-level training may lead to a reduced level of performance and possibly an injury.

After a race, take a complete rest from running (anything from two or three days for a 10K to a week or more for a marathon). This is a good time to cross-train. You can stay active, yet minimize any additional stress to your primary running muscles. The return to training should be gradual.

The success that runners report to us as a result of a carefully designed training program of quality training and quality recovery exemplifies the importance of balancing these two key training components. The following recovery plan was developed by my coauthor Scott Murr to guide marathoners through the post-race recovery process. After a race, many runners return to intense training too soon. Some are exhilarated with their performances and are committed to training even harder for even more improvement, while others are disappointed with their performances and jump back into training to seek redemption.

Here is the approach that we suggest to runners following a race.

POST-RACE RECOVERY

Marathon

THE WEEK AFTER A MARATHON	No running; maybe some light spinning or some swimming.
2 WEEKS AFTER A MARATHON	Light easy running, but when your body says "stop," you actually stop.
3 WEEKS AFTER A MARATHON	Back to some running, but absolutely no thoughts about distance or pace; listen to your body and energy level.
4 WEEKS AFTER A MARATHON	Back to a regular training routine, but without any focus on pace or effort.

Half-Marathon / 20K / 10-Miler / 15K

THE WEEK AFTER A RACE	Minimal running with some relaxed spinning and/or some swimming.
2 WEEKS AFTER A RACE	Back to some running without focus on pace or distance.
3 WEEKS AFTER A RACE	Back to a regular training routine, but intensity should be based on perceived effort rather than pace.

10K / 8K

THE WEEK AFTER A 10K / 8K   Some relaxed running, but intensity should be based on perceived effort rather than pace.

2 WEEKS AFTER A 10K / 8K   Back to a regular training routine, but intensity should be based on perceived effort rather than pace.

3 WEEKS AFTER A 10K / 8K   Back to a regular training routine.

5K

THE WEEK AFTER A 5K   Some relaxed running, but intensity should be based on perceived effort rather than pace.

2 WEEKS AFTER A 5K   Back to a regular training routine.

REAL RUNNER REPORT

February 4, 2014

Hi Bill and Scott,

I have been running for the last two years, and around October '13 adopted the 3plus2 program after buying the *Run Less Run Faster* book. I am 38 years old and reside in the city of Bangalore in India.

I followed the 16-week program for marathon and ended up with some very satisfying results! I ran my first marathon at the Standard Chartered Mumbai Marathon (SCMM) in January 2013 and had a time of 4 hours and 2 mins.

This January, in the SCMM 2014, I ended up with a time of 3 hours 34 mins after following the 16-week FIRST program. An astonishing 28 minutes off my personal best!

For me specifically, the training made a lot of sense and hope to follow this for the coming year as well!

Warm Regards,
Vijayaraghavan Venugopal
CEO, Fast & Up
Bangalore, India

January 21, 2015

Hi Bill,

It Is that time of the year when I come again to thank you and your team! At the SCMM 2015 marathon in Mumbai, held on January 18, I improved my timing from 3.34 to 3.24! My sole training guide in terms of planning the run/cross-training schedule for the last two years has been the *Run Less Run Faster* book.

Thank you and trust you are having great success training people all over the world!

Vijay

April 17, 2016

Hi Bill,

Hope you are doing great. I have been writing to you for the last two years on my development as a runner while with the RLRF program, which I follow in the latter half of every year. From a 3.34 at the Mumbai marathon in January 2014, I recently went under 3 hours (2:59:48) at the Paris marathon on April 3, 2016.

Going forward I hope to stay on the RLRF program and see how I can improve this a bit further.

Vijay

September 30, 2016

Hi Bill & Scott,

Once again some news to share—2:55 at Berlin Marathon. And now at the age of 41, the next stop is Boston.

Thanks for all those replies through the last few years!

Best Regards,
Vijay

PERFORMANCE FACTORS

9

Running Hot and Cold

When I awakened at 2:00 a.m. on the day of the Kiawah Island Marathon in December 2001, I realized that it was the sound of the condo's air-conditioning unit that roused me. Even in a half-awake state, I knew that was not good news for the marathon that would start in a few hours. At 5:00 a.m. I stepped out on the deck of the condo into the damp, warm conditions. My brother and I had traveled to Kiawah for its flat course with temperatures normally in the 50s in mid-December. We began a discussion about what to do—(1) forgo the marathon in the hot, humid conditions, (2) try to switch to the half-marathon, or (3) do part of the race as a training run.

We knew that we would not be able to match the 3:09 marathon that we had run in Pittsburgh on a hilly course in the late spring. Not in these conditions. We made the decision to modify our planned pace and proceed to the marathon starting line. Instead of running our planned pace of 7:13, we would compensate for the steamy conditions by relaxing our pace by 20 seconds per mile to 7:33. Over the last six miles of the marathon, we passed hundreds of runners and crossed the line in 3:18 with an overall pace of 7:33. Had we stuck with our original plan, we would have wilted like so many of the runners we had just passed. We knew that it was not possible to achieve our original marathon goal with the less-than-ideal 70-degree temperature. As it turns out, our 4% slower marathon provided the adjustment that still offered us a challenging, but attainable goal.

As any experienced runner knows, the weather is a critical factor in race performance. Months of excellent training can easily be undermined by high temperatures or humidity, a chilling headwind, or subfreezing temperatures. Before selecting a race, I check the 10-year weather history for the race city. However, averages can indicate only the likely temperature for a specific day. You make your race choice and hope that playing the percentages pays off. What do you do on those days that the unexpected occurs and the conditions are extreme? You have the option of not running the race and choosing another within the next couple of weeks. That choice will give you a chance to perform in conditions that are more conducive to achieving the goal finish time representative of your months of training. Another option is to run the race because it is one that you particularly want to experience. It may also be likely that you have incurred travel expenses, or arranged with friends to share the race experience. In that case, you must modify your goal finish time and your planned race pace, realizing that the conditions dictate the modification. The worst decision you can make is to believe that you can defy conditions and successfully run to your potential against the heat, wind, or extreme cold.

We receive an abundance of messages from runners in the southeastern USA or Southeast Asia, asking how to train in heat and humidity. In the western part of the United States, the low humidity and large daily range of temperature provide cooler times of day for workouts, reducing the chance of wilting. However, in the regions of the country with high humidity, it is not possible to run as fast in the summer months because of the challenging environmental conditions. So how should runners in these regions adjust their summer running?

There's no question that heat and humidity will slow your pace. This poses a problem for the runner who is using the summer months to prepare for a fall race. Because you will most likely not be running your fall marathon in the extreme heat and humidity that you will experience in the summer, training in very high temperatures—causing you to run 30 seconds per mile slower than your normal training pace—will not provide the preparation needed for that fall race.

To combat this problem, Scott Murr and I prepare during the summer for fall marathons by running early in the morning, when the temperatures are typically in the low 70s with little radiant heat, even though the humidity is high. There will still be a performance decrement, but the neuromuscular and biomechanical training will not be much different from fall training and racing. You can expect to run a little slower than your normal targeted pace. As long as your effort is challenging, but doable, you will be getting the benefits you are seeking. Running in the afternoons with a 90+ degree heat index does not permit the faster running needed for training specificity, at least not safely.

We recognize that our location in the western part of the Carolinas provides cooler temperatures than those near the coast or those in the deep South, where temperatures can be in the 80s or even 90s in early morning. For those runners, it makes sense to choose a late-fall race so that they have time to perform long training runs in early fall with cooler temperatures. In Chapter 6, we discussed using a treadmill for performing runs at a faster pace than what is possible outside. The lower temperature and humidity of the indoor environment will enable you to run at a faster pace than the outdoor heat would permit. Mixing outdoor running for acclimatization with indoor running for speed may be a good race preparation strategy. Consider the specificity principle. Try to train in conditions similar to those you will be racing in.

Both an increase in air temperature and increased metabolic activity challenge a runner's capacity for controlling core temperature. A runner is cooled as sweat evaporates from the skin. Humid conditions, characterized by a relatively high level of water vapor, slow the rate of evaporation of sweat from the skin. Thus, little or no cooling occurs. Without any evaporative cooling, more stress is placed on the circulatory system to carry heat from the working muscles to the surface of the skin, where the heat is transferred to the air surrounding the skin. As the body attempts to carry away the heat, heart rate increases to move more blood to the surface. Because body temperature is not being cooled by evaporation, the body is signaled to increase the sweat rate, which reduces blood volume and adds to the stress on the circulatory system. This stressful sequence illustrates the problems created for a runner in very humid conditions, and shows why runners need to adjust their intensity in those situations.

Table 9.2 provides an estimate of how climatic conditions affect your training and racing. As described in the previous paragraph, high humidity creates major cooling problems during intense physical activity. Two methods of assessing humid conditions include relative humidity and dew point. Relative humidity is the percentage of water vapor in the air at a given temperature. The dew point is the temperature in which there is 100 percent water vapor in the air. There are tables that use temperature and relative humidity for assessing the hazards of running by calculating a heat index. There are also tables that use temperature and the dew point for assessing the hazards of running by summing those two values. FIRST has chosen to use the temperature and dew point to determine the effects of the climatic conditions on the training paces and race times of runners.

TABLE 9.1

Adjust Running for Heat and Humidity

TEMPERATURE + DEW POINT	ADJUSTMENT
110 or less	No Adjustment
120	1%
130	2%
140	3%
150	4.5%
160	6%
170	8%
180	10%
Greater than 180	Stay inside

TABLE 9.2

Adjusted 5K Times for Heat and Humidity

5K-time	Adjusted 5K Time						
	1%	2%	3%	4.5%	6%	8%	10%
16:00	16:10	16:19	16:29	16:43	16:58	17:17	17:36
16:10	16:20	16:29	16:39	16:54	17:08	17:28	17:47
16:20	16:30	16:40	16:49	17:04	17:19	17:38	17:58
16:30	16:40	16:50	17:00	17:15	17:29	17:49	18:09
16:40	16:50	17:00	17:10	17:25	17:40	18:00	18:20
16:50	17:00	17:10	17:20	17:34	17:51	18:11	18:31
17:00	17:10	17:20	17:31	17:46	18:01	18:22	18:42
17:10	17:20	17:31	17:41	17:56	18:12	18:32	18:53
17:20	17:30	17:41	17:51	18:07	18:22	18:43	19:04
17:30	17:41	17:51	18:02	18:17	18:33	18:54	19:15
17:40	17:51	18:01	18:12	18:28	18:44	19:05	19:26
17:50	18:01	18:11	18:22	18:38	18:54	19:16	19:37
18:00	18:11	18:22	18:32	18:49	19:05	19:26	19:48
18:10	18:21	18:32	18:43	18:59	19:15	19:37	19:59
18:20	18:31	18:42	18:53	19:10	19:26	19:48	20:10
18:30	18:41	18:52	19:03	19:20	19:37	19:59	20:21
18:40	18:51	19:02	19:14	19:30	19:47	20:10	20:32
18:50	19:01	19:13	19:24	19:41	19:58	20:20	20:43
19:00	19:11	19:23	19:34	19:51	20:08	20:31	20:54
19:10	19:22	19:33	19:45	20:02	20:19	20:42	21:05
19:20	19:32	19:43	19:55	20:12	20:30	20:53	21:16
19:30	19:42	19:53	20:05	20:23	20:40	21:04	21:27
19:40	19:52	20:04	20:15	20:33	20:51	21:14	21:38
19:50	20:02	20:14	20:26	20:44	21:01	21:26	21:49
20:00	20:12	20:24	20:36	20:54	21:12	21:36	22:00
20:10	20:22	20:34	20:46	21:04	21:23	21:47	22:11
20:20	20:32	20:44	20:57	21:15	21:33	21:58	22:22
20:30	20:42	20:55	21:07	21:25	21:44	22:08	22:33
20:40	20:52	21:05	21:17	21:36	21:54	22:19	22:44
20:50	21:03	21:15	21:28	21:46	22:05	22:30	22:55

5K-time	Adjusted 5K Time						
	1%	2%	3%	4.5%	6%	8%	10%
21:00	21:13	21:25	21:38	21:57	22:16	22:41	23:06
21:10	21:23	21:35	21:48	22:07	22:26	22:52	23:17
21:20	21:33	21:46	21:58	22:18	22:37	23:02	23:28
21:30	21:43	21:56	22:09	22:28	22:48	23:13	23:39
21:40	21:53	22:06	22:19	22:39	22:58	23:24	23:50
21:50	22:03	22:16	22:29	22:49	23:09	23:35	24:01
22:00	22:13	22:26	22:40	22:59	23:19	23:46	24:12
22:10	22:23	22:37	22:50	23:10	23:30	23:56	24:23
22:20	22:33	22:47	23:00	23:20	23:40	24:07	24:34
22:30	22:44	22:57	23:11	23:31	23:51	24:18	24:45
22:40	22:54	23:07	23:21	23:41	24:02	24:29	24:56
22:50	23:04	23:17	23:31	23:52	24:12	24:40	25:07
23:00	23:14	23:28	23:41	24:02	24:23	24:50	25:18
23:10	23:24	23:38	23:54	24:13	24:33	25:01	25:29
23:20	23:34	23:48	24:02	24:23	24:44	25:12	25:40
23:30	23:44	23:58	24:12	24:33	24:55	25:23	25:51
23:40	23:54	24:08	24:23	24:44	25:05	25:34	26:02
23:50	24:04	24:19	24:33	24:54	25:16	25:44	26:13
24:00	24:14	24:29	24:43	25:05	25:26	25:55	26:24
24:10	24:25	24:39	24:54	25:15	25:37	26:06	26:35
24:20	24:35	24:49	25:04	25:26	25:48	26:17	26:46
24:30	24:45	24:59	25:14	25:36	25:58	26:28	26:57
24:40	24:55	25:10	25:24	25:47	26:09	26:38	27:08
24:50	25:05	25:20	25:35	25:57	26:19	26:49	27:19
25:00	25:15	25:30	25:45	26:08	26:30	27:00	27:30
25:10	25:25	25:40	25:55	26:18	26:41	27:11	27:41
25:20	25:35	25:50	26:06	26:28	26:51	27:22	27:52
25:30	25:45	26:01	26:16	26:39	27:02	27:32	28:03
25:40	25:55	26:11	26:26	26:49	27:12	27:43	28:14
25:50	26:06	26:21	26:37	27:00	27:23	27:54	28:25
26:00	26:16	26:31	26:47	27:10	27:34	28:05	28:36
26:10	26:26	26:41	26:57	27:21	27:44	28:16	28:47

5K-time	Adjusted 5K Time						
	1%	2%	3%	4.5%	6%	8%	10%
26:20	26:36	26:52	27:07	27:31	27:55	28:26	28:58
26:30	26:46	27:02	27:18	27:42	28:05	28:37	29:09
26:40	26:56	27:12	27:28	27:52	28:16	28:48	29:20
26:50	27:06	27:22	27:38	28:02	28:27	28:59	29:31
27:00	27:16	27:32	27:49	28:13	28:37	29:10	29:42
27:10	27:26	27:43	27:59	28:23	28:48	29:20	29:53
27:20	27:36	27:53	28:09	28:34	28:58	29:31	30:04
27:30	27:47	28:03	28:20	28:44	29:09	29:42	30:15
27:40	27:57	28:13	28:30	28:55	29:20	29:53	30:26
27:50	28:07	28:23	28:40	29:05	29:30	30:04	30:37
28:00	28:17	28:34	28:50	29:16	29:41	30:14	30:48
28:10	28:27	28:44	29:01	29:26	29:51	30:25	30:59
28:20	28:37	28:54	29:11	29:37	30:02	30:36	31:10
28:30	28:47	29:04	29:21	29:47	30:13	30:47	31:21
28:40	28:57	29:14	29:32	29:57	30:23	30:58	31:32
28:50	29:07	29:25	29:42	30:08	30:34	31:08	31:43
29:00	29:17	29:35	29:52	30:18	30:44	31:19	31:54
29:10	29:28	29:45	30:03	30:29	30:55	31:30	32:05
29:20	29:38	29:55	30:13	30:39	31:06	31:41	32:16
29:30	29:48	30:05	30:23	30:50	31:16	31:52	32:27
29:40	29:58	30:16	30:33	31:00	31:27	32:02	32:38
29:50	30:08	30:26	30:44	31:11	31:37	32:13	32:49
30:00	30:18	30:36	30:54	31:21	31:48	32:24	33:00
30:10	30:28	30:46	31:04	31:31	31:59	32:35	33:11
30:20	30:38	30:56	31:15	31:42	32:09	32:46	33:22
30:30	30:48	31:07	31:25	31:52	32:20	32:56	33:33
30:40	30:58	31:17	31:35	32:03	32:30	33:07	33:44
30:50	31:09	31:27	31:46	32:13	32:41	33:18	33:55
31:00	31:19	31:37	31:56	32:24	32:52	33:29	34:06
31:10	31:29	31:47	32:06	32:34	33:02	33:40	34:17
31:20	31:39	31:58	32:16	32:45	33:13	33:50	34:28
31:30	31:49	32:08	32:27	32:55	33:23	34:01	34:39

	Adjusted 5K Time						
5K-time	1%	2%	3%	4.5%	6%	8%	10%
31:40	31:59	32:18	32:37	33:06	33:34	34:12	34:50
31:50	32:09	32:28	32:47	33:16	33:45	34:23	35:01
32:00	32:19	32:38	32:58	33:26	33:55	34:34	35:12
32:10	32:29	32:49	33:08	33:37	34:06	34:44	35:23
32:20	32:39	32:59	33:18	33:47	34:16	34:55	35:34
32:30	32:50	33:09	33:29	33:58	34:27	35:06	35:45
32:40	33:00	33:19	33:39	34:08	34:38	35:17	35:56
32:50	33:10	33:29	33:49	34:19	34:48	35:28	36:07
33:00	33:20	33:40	33:59	34:29	34:59	35:38	36:18
33:10	33:30	33:50	34:10	34:40	35:09	35:49	36:29
33:20	33:40	34:00	34:20	34:50	35:20	36:00	36:40
33:30	33:50	34:10	34:30	35:00	35:31	36:11	36:51
33:40	34:00	34:20	34:41	35:11	35:41	36:22	37:02
33:50	34:10	34:31	34:51	35:21	35:52	36:32	37:13
34:00	34:20	34:41	35:01	35:32	36:02	36:43	37:24
34:10	34:31	34:51	35:12	35:42	36:13	36:54	37:35
34:20	34:41	35:01	35:22	35:53	36:24	37:05	37:46
34:30	34:51	35:11	35:32	36:03	36:34	37:16	37:57
34:40	35:01	35:22	35:42	36:14	36:45	37:26	38:08
34:50	35:11	35:32	35:53	36:24	36:55	37:37	38:19
35:00	35:21	35:42	36:03	36:35	37:06	37:48	38:30
35:10	35:31	35:52	36:13	36:45	37:17	37:59	38:41
35:20	35:41	36:02	36:24	36:55	37:27	38:10	38:52
35:30	35:51	36:13	36:34	37:06	37:38	38:20	39:03
35:40	36:01	36:23	36:44	37:16	37:48	38:31	39:14
35:50	36:12	36:33	36:55	37:27	37:59	38:42	39:25
36:00	36:22	36:43	37:05	37:37	38:10	38:53	39:36
36:10	36:32	36:53	37:15	37:48	38:20	39:04	39:47
36:20	36:42	37:04	37:25	37:58	38:31	39:14	39:58
36:30	36:52	37:14	37:36	38:09	38:41	39:25	40:09
36:40	37:02	37:24	37:46	38:19	38:52	39:36	40:20
36:50	37:12	37:34	37:56	38:29	39:03	39:47	40:31

			Adjusted 5K Time				
5K-time	1%	2%	3%	4.5%	6%	8%	10%
37:00	37:22	37:44	38:07	38:40	39:13	39:58	40:42
37:10	37:32	37:55	38:17	38:50	39:24	40:08	40:53
37:20	37:42	38:05	38:27	39:01	39:34	40:19	41:04
37:30	37:53	38:15	38:38	39:11	39:45	40:30	41:15
37:40	38:03	38:25	38:48	39:22	39:56	40:41	41:26
37:50	38:13	38:35	38:58	39:32	40:06	40:52	41:37
38:00	38:23	38:46	39:08	39:43	40:17	41:02	41:48
38:10	38:33	38:56	39:19	39:53	40:27	41:13	41:59
38:20	38:43	39:06	39:29	40:04	40:38	41:24	42:10
38:30	38:53	39:16	39:39	40:14	40:49	41:35	42:21
38:40	39:03	39:26	39:50	40:24	40:59	41:46	42:32
38:50	39:13	39:37	40:00	40:35	41:10	41:56	42:43
39:00	39:23	39:47	40:10	40:45	41:20	42:07	42:54
39:10	39:34	39:57	40:21	40:56	41:31	42:18	43:05
39:20	39:44	40:07	40:31	41:06	41:42	42:29	43:16
39:30	39:54	40:17	40:41	41:17	41:52	42:40	43:27
39:40	40:04	40:28	40:51	41:27	42:03	42:50	43:38
39:50	40:14	40:38	41:02	41:38	42:13	43:01	43:49
40:00	40:24	40:48	41:12	41:48	42:24	43:12	44:00

Here is how to use Tables 9.1 and 9.2 to adjust training paces and race times according to the temperature and dew point.

- Add the temperature and the dew point. Both numbers are easily found on most weather websites.

- Find the corresponding percentage adjustment in Table 9.1.

- Go to Table 9.2 and find the percentage adjustment on the top of the table. Look across the row from your 5K time and find the adjusted 5K time in the column under the percentage adjustment, based on the sum of your temperature and dew point.

- Use the adjusted 5K time for selecting the target times and paces for your three Key Runs.

- Use your weather-adjusted 5K time for determining a more realistic race target, given the weather conditions on race day. Go to Table 3.1 and use the adjusted 5K time to find the corresponding 10K, half-marathon, and marathon predicted times.

Running Hot and Cold: Q & A

Q. *What is a hot environment?*

A. If you are a runner, when the temperature begins to climb over 60°F, you can expect the temperature to influence your running; that is, a 1–2% increase in metabolic cost for each 1.5°F increase in temperature. This performance decrement becomes more pronounced as the race distance increases. Add increased humidity to an already warm day and the impact on your running is even more pronounced. Your expected performance goals must be adjusted when you encounter high temperatures and humidity.

Q. *How important is hydration in countering the effects of heat?*

A. Very important. The answer to this question could easily be an entire chapter. You must be aware that hydration becomes a key factor in running performance in those sessions lasting more than one hour. A 2–3% water loss will result in a significant performance decrement. However, staying hydrated does not offset the increased metabolic and physiological stress associated with higher environmental temperatures. Also important to note: Wet skin does not sweat as much (and cool you down as much) as dry skin. Therefore, "Pour it in, don't pour it on." In other words, drink water rather than pouring it on top of your head.

Q. *How can you be sure you are drinking enough, but not too much?*

A. Make sure that your urine output is plentiful and the color is clear or pale yellow before you begin your run. If you are losing more than 1.5% of your body weight during a run, you are losing too much fluid through sweat and need to drink more before and during your run.

Q. *How do you acclimatize to the heat?*

A. Heat acclimatization requires exercising in the heat. Simply sitting in a hot environment, even for extended periods, will not result in the adaptations necessary for exercising in the heat. The body learns to sweat more effectively and to tolerate liquid replacement as you train in hot environments. The body requires 10–14 days for complete acclimatization to elevated environmental temperatures, although initial adaptations occur in the first five days of acclimatization.

Q. *What's a runner to do when it's hot?*

A. You will not be able to sustain as fast a pace as normal in the heat, even after adequate acclimatization. In Key Run #1, you may substitute short repeats (400s, 800s) for longer repeats (1200s, 1600s). Another strategy that can be utilized in the heat is to take longer recoveries between repeats and hydrate throughout the workout. In Key Runs #2 and #3, you may not be able to maintain the prescribed pace for the specified distance. Run the specified distance at an effort you perceive as moderate to hard. When running in hot, humid conditions, be smart and listen to your body.

Q. *How do I know if I am experiencing a heat disorder and what should I do?*

A. There are three major categories of heat injury: heat cramps, heat exhaustion, and heat stroke. Heat cramps, the mildest form of heat disorder, are painful, involuntary muscle spasms. Heat exhaustion may include muscle cramps along with excessive sweating, weak pulse, dizziness, and a headache. Heat stroke, the most severe heat disorder, is marked by a high fever, sweating cessation, and may include unconsciousness. It should be treated as a medical emergency. All these conditions can be prevented with proper fluid intake and by paying appropriate attention to the common symptoms associated with heat disorders. Heat injuries can be serious. It is important to listen to your body and train smart. It is not necessary to risk your health to complete a run just because it is on your schedule.

Q. *What are the risks associated with exercising in the cold?*

A. Exercise in cold environments presents few risks to the runner who does proper preparation. Generally, even in cold weather, the significant amount of heat produced as a result of exercise will more than maintain core temperature. Only after extended exercise with the depletion of glycogen stores and the resultant fatigue will there be a risk that the body does not produce enough heat to maintain a sufficient core temperature. At that time, the risk of hypothermia can become a concern.

You must pay close attention to dress, hydration, length of race, and energy sources. As long as you generate more heat than you lose, exercising in the cold should not present the problems that exercising in the heat does.

Q. *How should the runner dress for cold weather?*

A. We wish we could create easy-to-use tables for choosing racing gear for every 10°F interval. However, while many runners are comfortable in a short-sleeved T-shirt at 40°F, some want a long-sleeved tee anytime the temperature drops below 50°F. My fingers and toes are unusually sensitive to the cold, and you'll find me with ski mittens while others aren't even wearing cotton gloves.

Even with the wide variation in individuals' tolerance for cold, there are some general guidelines we find useful. The most important is to remain dry while keeping warm. Adding layers of clothing as the temperature drops and/or the wind picks up is usually the most effective way to keep moisture away from your body. The layer next to your body should be a material that wicks moisture away from your skin. Silk will accomplish that, as will a number of high-tech synthetic materials. Even when you are only wearing a T-shirt, it's a good idea to keep the moisture away from your skin. Remember: You perspire constantly and the rate of sweating picks up as you exercise more strenuously.

You may need to add a second layer of insulating material, such as wool, down, or fleece if you need to keep your body heat in. Finally, you may need to add a wind- and water-resistant shell to protect yourself from the elements, if you are running in severe conditions. This layer should be capable of letting moisture pass outward. The advantage to using layering is that you can peel off unneeded clothing if conditions improve or if your body provides sufficient heat to keep you feeling warm without the need for an insulating layer.

Once the temperature is below freezing, and especially if there is much wind, you must be aware that frostbite can affect your extremities. Gloves are fine, but mittens conserve more heat. Remember to cover your head, since a great deal of heat is lost through the head. Finally, socks that wick moisture are just as important for cold weather running as they are for hot weather running. Your feet produce great amounts of moisture that need to be eliminated. Breathable shoes will complement high-tech wicking socks.

Q. *Is hydration important in cold weather?*

A. Most individuals tend to take in less liquid when they are exposed to a cold environment, even when exercising. Just as in the heat, thirst is a very poor measure of your need for fluids.

Fluid replacement in a cold environment is important, but it typically is not as obvious to the runner as it is in warm conditions.

Q. *What's a runner to do when it is cold?*

A. Follow the guidelines above and be prepared to be uncomfortably cold for the first 10 minutes of your run. If you are comfortable when you start your run in the cold, you will be too hot once you begin producing heat. It is well worth the expense of purchasing technical clothing that wicks away moisture. You can remain remarkably dry while running. Not having wet clothes against your skin makes all the difference in your ability to stay warm and have a pleasant run.

When checking the temperature to determine how many layers

to wear for your run, don't neglect to check the windchill. Wind-chill better reflects "real feel." It is nice to have an outer layer that can be zipped and unzipped as you move into a headwind or a tail-wind. And don't forget the sunscreen just because it is cold!

|||||| ▬▬▬▬▬▬▬▬▬▬▬▬▬▬▬▬▬▬▬▬▬▬

REAL RUNNER REPORT

To: Bill Pierce
Subject: Thank you for an amazing program

I just wanted to write in thanks for your amazing running program. I am 38 and started getting more into my running about five years ago when my youngest daughter started school. I started learning about your program about four years ago and I love it. It is a perfect fit for my lifestyle.

I just had some great PRs in four different distances in the last year with a marathon yesterday in 3:03, a half-marathon in the fall in 1:27, a 5K last summer in 18:55, and a 10K in the fall in 38:40. It really works! I'm hoping I can keep improving before I get too old. :)

Thank you,
Katie Renz
Industrial Engineer (currently a stay-at-home mom)
Appleton, Wisconsin

▬▬▬▬▬▬▬▬▬▬▬▬▬▬▬▬▬▬▬▬▬▬ ||||||

10

Altitude Training and Racing

It's fun to travel around the country and around the globe to races at interesting and scenic destinations. Some of my most memorable runs occurred in Colorado, Utah, and Idaho. Living in the foothills of the Blue Ridge Mountains in South Carolina, I could not readily prepare to race at elevations between 6,000 and 9,000 feet. FIRST often receives messages from runners asking how to prepare for a race at high altitude, as well as requests from runners living in the high country of the West asking what they can expect when running at sea level based on their training paces and race times in higher elevations.

Runners living in the high elevations of the Rocky Mountains—Denver (5,280 feet), Aspen (8,000 feet), Laramie (7,200 feet)—often travel to lower-elevation marathons hoping to qualify for the Boston Marathon. They believe the benefits of living in the rarefied mountain air will make running in the denser sea-level air a breeze and sweep them to a qualifying time not attainable in the high mountains. Similarly, runners living in the low country on the East or West Coasts want to know how to prepare for a race in the high country of the West. How do they adjust their finish time expectations?

Even though individuals react differently to the challenges presented by the thinner air, this chapter provides general guidelines for how to adjust training under these taxing conditions. In particular, we have included a table for how those living in the high country can adjust their training for races at sea level and how those living at lower elevations should adjust their race goals for high-elevation races.

The Challenges of Living High/Racing Low and Living Low/Racing High

It has long been thought that training at a higher elevation with its thinner air and the resultant inadequate oxygen supply would provide an advantage to runners when they return to sea level for a race. Because the lower atmospheric pressure at high elevations makes blood less oxygen-rich, it stimulates the body's production of red blood cell volume. This, in turn, increases the availability of hemoglobin, the oxygen-carrying pigment and predominant protein in red blood cells. The resultant increased capability of delivering more oxygen to the working muscles contributes to an improvement in aerobic capacity (VO_2 max), a prime determinant of endurance performance. Studies have shown that living and sleeping at elevations greater than 7,000 feet produce these physiological changes. However, these physiological adaptations do not necessarily translate into an improved performance or faster running times. Why is that?

The thinner air at higher elevations slows running performance. Race times at high elevations are much slower than at sea level. World-class competitions at high elevations, as demonstrated at the 1968 Olympics in Mexico City (7,382 feet above sea level), produce much slower times for races greater than 800 meters. It is common for teams to move to higher elevations to acclimatize their bodies to the thinner air before going to a competition being held at high elevation. That's what the USA track team did in 1968 when they set up training camp near South Lake Tahoe (7,300 feet elevation) prior to the Olympic Games in Mexico City.

The primary limitation on enhancing running performance at sea level by altitude training is that runners cannot train at as fast a pace at altitude as they could at sea level. Losing the ability to train at sea-level speed generally offsets the benefits gained from the increased physiological adaptations. A 1997 study investigated how the benefits of living at high elevations could translate to improved performances when a runner returned to a lower elevation.[1] Three groups of elite runners were placed in different scenarios for four weeks—one group lived, slept, and trained at an elevation greater than 8,000 feet (HH); another group lived and slept at the same high elevation, but trained below 4,000 feet (HL); and a third group lived, slept, and trained at an elevation below 4,000 feet (LL). While both the live high and train high (HH) group, and the live high, train low (HL) group had increased red blood cell volumes and concomitant VO_2 max increases, it was only the HL group that had improved 5K race times in a low-elevation race. The LL group did not show any improvement in physiological measures or race times.

What can be learned from this study is that the physiological benefits of living and sleeping at a high altitude need to be accompanied by an opportunity to train at a lower elevation. That permits sea-level training paces to be maintained, along with neuromuscular patterns of fast running. Studies also show that the physiological benefits from training high can only be maintained for two to three weeks following a runner's return to a lower elevation. Timing your training along with your targeted races must be carefully planned.

Additionally, studies show that individual differences in response to altitude training vary.[2] There are high responders to the high altitude, low responders, and non-responders.[3] Therefore, individuals must experiment to determine how they respond to temporary moves to a high elevation in their pursuit of aerobic benefits.

Can High-Elevation Running Conditions Be Simulated at Lower Elevations?

Some companies market altitude-simulation systems to be used overnight. They claim that these systems simulate sleeping at high altitude, which stimulates the beneficial physiological adaptations (like increased red blood cells) acquired by living at high altitude.

Similarly, there are companies marketing altitude masks that runners can wear while training. Their claim is that this hypoxic training simulates training at high altitude by reducing the availability of oxygen.

These methods do not simulate the conditions of living or training at a high elevation.[4] Basically, these types of products make breathing more difficult by reducing the amount of oxygen available in inspired air. Nitrogen, which comprises 78 percent of atmospheric air, is substituted for oxygen to reduce the percentage of oxygen in the air that is being breathed (atmospheric air is 20.95% oxygen). At a high elevation, the percentage of oxygen in the air is the same as at sea level (20.95%). It is the lower atmospheric pressure that reduces the partial pressure of oxygen that makes oxygen less available. While the marketing may be persuasive, there is no strong evidence that these products will produce the desired physiological changes or produce faster performance times.

How to Adjust Running Paces at High Elevations

Runners living in the Western states with elevations 5,000 feet and greater encounter the limitations on distance running associated with running in thin air. The most common question we receive is how runners should adjust training target times and paces for the three Key Runs if they live in Albuquerque, Flagstaff, Laramie, Park City, or other high-country locations in order to prepare for a running performance target at sea level. While individuals may have different abilities to cope with the physiological effects from the thinner air, we have developed a table that shows how to adjust times and paces to sea-level equivalencies.

The NCAA permits adjustments to qualifying times for regional and national competitions for races run at high elevations. From these guidelines, we developed a table that provides runners with adjusted training paces at altitude to prepare them for racing at sea level. Conversely, the table can be used by a sea-level runner to select an appropriate race time goal for a race at altitude.

Here's an example of how we can use Table 10.1 to advise runners on how to train for a marathon at sea level when they live at altitude. A request came from three women living and training in Santa Fe, New Mexico (an elevation of 7,000 feet), who wanted to know how they could use the FIRST Training Program to train for running a 3:30 marathon in New York City. I knew that they could not expect to run FIRST's target paces designated for the 3:30 marathon. Here's how I determined the appropriate training level at 7,000 feet for a specific sea-level goal:

- I went to Table 3.1 and found the equivalent 5K time for a 3:30 marathon goal, which was 21:35.

- Next, I used Table 10.1 to find the equivalent 5K time at 7,000 feet for a sea-level 5K time of 21:35, which was 22:35.

- I recommended that they use the adjusted 5K time of 22:35 for selecting the training paces for the three Key Runs (Tables 6.6–6.8) for the FIRST Marathon Training Plan (Table 6.5).

If the runners were able to run a 22:35 5K in Santa Fe at an elevation of 7,000 feet, where they would do their training, then a 3:30 marathon at sea level would be realistic, given the benefit of training high but racing low. They confirmed that the training times and paces were challenging, but realistic. All three achieved their 3:30 goals in New York.

TABLE 10.1

ELEVATION-ADJUSTED 5K TIMES

SEA LEVEL 5K-time	FEET ABOVE SEA LEVEL										
	2000	3000	3500	4000	4500	5000	5500	6000	6500	7000	7500
16:00	16:09	16:12	16:16	16:18	16:24	16:28	16:32	16:35	16:40	16:46	16:52
16:10	16:19	16:22	16:26	16:28	16:34	16:38	16:43	16:45	16:50	16:56	17:03
16:20	16:29	16:33	16:36	16:38	16:44	16:48	16:53	16:56	17:01	17:06	17:13
16:30	16:39	16:43	16:47	16:49	16:54	16:58	17:03	17:06	17:11	17:17	17:24
16:40	16:49	16:53	16:57	16:59	17:05	17:09	17:14	17:17	17:22	17:27	17:34
16:50	16:59	17:03	17:07	17:09	17:15	17:19	17:24	17:27	17:32	17:38	17:45
17:00	17:09	17:13	17:17	17:19	17:25	17:29	17:34	17:37	17:42	17:48	17:55
17:10	17:19	17:23	17:27	17:29	17:35	17:40	17:45	17:48	17:53	17:59	18:06
17:20	17:29	17:33	17:37	17:40	17:46	17:50	17:55	17:58	18:03	18:09	18:17
17:30	17:39	17:43	17:48	17:50	17:56	18:00	18:05	18:08	18:14	18:20	18:27
17:40	17:49	17:54	17:58	18:00	18:06	18:10	18:16	18:19	18:24	18:30	18:38
17:50	18:00	18:04	18:08	18:10	18:16	18:21	18:26	18:29	18:34	18:41	18:48
18:00	18:10	18:14	18:18	18:20	18:27	18:31	18:36	18:39	18:45	18:51	18:59
18:10	18:20	18:24	18:28	18:30	18:37	18:41	18:47	18:50	18:55	19:02	19:09
18:20	18:30	18:34	18:38	18:41	18:47	18:52	18:57	19:00	19:06	19:12	19:20
18:30	18:40	18:44	18:49	18:51	18:57	19:02	19:07	19:11	19:16	19:23	19:30
18:40	18:50	18:54	18:59	19:01	19:08	19:12	19:18	19:21	19:26	19:33	19:41

SEA LEVEL 5K-time	FEET ABOVE SEA LEVEL										
	2000	3000	3500	4000	4500	5000	5500	6000	6500	7000	7500
18:50	19:00	19:05	19:09	19:11	19:18	19:22	19:28	19:31	19:37	19:44	19:51
19:00	19:10	19:15	19:19	19:21	19:28	19:33	19:38	19:42	19:47	19:54	20:02
19:10	19:20	19:25	19:29	19:32	19:38	19:43	19:49	19:52	19:58	20:05	20:12
19:20	19:30	19:35	19:39	19:42	19:49	19:53	19:59	20:02	20:08	20:15	20:23
19:30	19:40	19:45	19:50	19:52	19:59	20:04	20:09	20:13	20:19	20:25	20:34
19:40	19:50	19:55	20:00	20:02	20:09	20:14	20:20	20:23	20:29	20:36	20:44
19:50	20:01	20:05	20:10	20:12	20:19	20:24	20:30	20:34	20:39	20:46	20:55
20:00	20:11	20:15	20:20	20:23	20:30	20:34	20:40	20:44	20:50	20:57	21:05
20:10	20:21	20:26	20:30	20:33	20:40	20:45	20:51	20:54	21:00	21:07	21:16
20:20	20:31	20:36	20:40	20:43	20:50	20:55	21:01	21:05	21:11	21:18	21:26
20:30	20:41	20:46	20:51	20:53	21:00	21:05	21:11	21:15	21:21	21:28	21:37
20:40	20:51	20:56	21:01	21:03	21:11	21:16	21:22	21:25	21:31	21:39	21:47
20:50	21:01	21:06	21:11	21:13	21:21	21:26	21:32	21:36	21:42	21:49	21:58
21:00	21:11	21:16	21:21	21:24	21:31	21:36	21:42	21:46	21:52	22:00	22:08
21:10	21:21	21:26	21:31	21:34	21:41	21:46	21:53	21:56	22:03	22:10	22:19
21:20	21:31	21:36	21:42	21:44	21:52	21:57	22:03	22:07	22:13	22:21	22:30
21:30	21:41	21:47	21:52	21:54	22:02	22:07	22:13	22:17	22:24	22:31	22:40
21:40	21:52	21:57	22:02	22:04	22:12	22:17	22:24	22:28	22:34	22:42	22:51
21:50	22:02	22:07	22:12	22:15	22:22	22:28	22:34	22:38	22:44	22:52	23:01
22:00	22:12	22:17	22:22	22:25	22:33	22:38	22:44	22:48	22:55	23:03	23:12
22:10	22:22	22:27	22:32	22:35	22:43	22:48	22:55	22:59	23:05	23:13	23:22
22:20	22:32	22:37	22:43	22:45	22:53	22:58	23:05	23:09	23:16	23:24	23:33
22:30	22:42	22:47	22:53	22:55	23:03	23:09	23:15	23:19	23:26	23:34	23:43
22:40	22:52	22:57	23:03	23:06	23:14	23:19	23:26	23:30	23:36	23:45	23:54
22:50	23:02	23:08	23:13	23:16	23:24	23:29	23:36	23:40	23:47	23:55	24:04
23:00	23:12	23:18	23:23	23:26	23:34	23:40	23:46	23:50	23:57	24:05	24:15
23:10	23:22	23:28	23:33	23:36	23:44	23:50	23:57	24:01	24:08	24:16	24:26
23:20	23:32	23:38	23:44	23:46	23:55	24:00	24:07	24:11	24:18	24:26	24:36
23:30	23:43	23:48	23:54	23:56	24:05	24:10	24:17	24:22	24:29	24:37	24:47
23:40	23:53	23:58	24:04	24:07	24:15	24:21	24:28	24:32	24:39	24:47	24:57
23:50	24:03	24:08	24:14	24:17	24:25	24:31	24:38	24:42	24:49	24:58	25:08
24:00	24:13	24:18	24:24	24:27	24:36	24:41	24:48	24:53	25:00	25:08	25:18
24:10	24:23	24:29	24:34	24:37	24:46	24:52	24:59	25:03	25:10	25:19	25:29

SEA LEVEL 5K-time	FEET ABOVE SEA LEVEL										
	2000	3000	3500	4000	4500	5000	5500	6000	6500	7000	7500
24:20	24:33	24:39	24:45	24:47	24:56	25:02	25:09	25:13	25:21	25:29	25:39
24:30	24:43	24:49	24:55	24:58	25:06	25:12	25:19	25:24	25:31	25:40	25:50
24:40	24:53	24:59	25:05	25:08	25:17	25:22	25:30	25:34	25:41	25:50	26:00
24:50	25:03	25:09	25:15	25:18	25:27	25:33	25:40	25:44	25:52	26:01	26:11
25:00	25:13	25:19	25:25	25:28	25:37	25:43	25:50	25:55	26:02	26:11	26:22
25:10	25:23	25:29	25:35	25:38	25:47	25:53	26:01	26:05	26:13	26:22	26:32
25:20	25:34	25:40	25:46	25:49	25:58	26:04	26:11	26:16	26:23	26:32	26:43
25:30	25:44	25:50	25:56	25:59	26:08	26:14	26:21	26:26	26:33	26:43	26:53
25:40	25:54	26:00	26:06	26:09	26:18	26:24	26:32	26:36	26:44	26:53	27:04
25:50	26:04	26:10	26:16	26:19	26:28	26:34	26:42	26:47	26:54	27:04	27:14
26:00	26:14	26:20	26:26	26:29	26:39	26:45	26:52	26:57	27:05	27:14	27:25
26:10	26:24	26:30	26:36	26:39	26:49	26:55	27:03	27:07	27:15	27:24	27:35
26:20	26:34	26:40	26:47	26:50	26:59	27:05	27:13	27:18	27:26	27:35	27:46
26:30	26:44	26:50	26:57	27:00	27:09	27:16	27:23	27:28	27:36	27:45	27:56
26:40	26:54	27:01	27:07	27:10	27:20	27:26	27:34	27:38	27:46	27:56	28:07
26:50	27:04	27:11	27:17	27:20	27:30	27:36	27:44	27:49	27:57	28:06	28:18
27:00	27:14	27:21	27:27	27:30	27:40	27:46	27:54	27:59	28:07	28:17	28:28
27:10	27:24	27:31	27:37	27:41	27:50	27:57	28:05	28:10	28:18	28:27	28:39
27:20	27:35	27:41	27:48	27:51	28:01	28:07	28:15	28:20	28:28	28:38	28:49
27:30	27:45	27:51	27:58	28:01	28:11	28:17	28:25	28:30	28:38	28:48	29:00
27:40	27:55	28:01	28:08	28:11	28:21	28:28	28:36	28:41	28:49	28:59	29:10
27:50	28:05	28:11	28:18	28:21	28:31	28:38	28:46	28:51	28:59	29:09	29:21
28:00	28:15	28:22	28:28	28:32	28:42	28:48	28:56	29:01	29:10	29:20	29:31
28:10	28:25	28:32	28:38	28:42	28:52	28:58	29:07	29:12	29:20	29:30	29:42
28:20	28:35	28:42	28:49	28:52	29:02	29:09	29:17	29:22	29:31	29:41	29:52
28:30	28:45	28:52	28:59	29:02	29:12	29:19	29:27	29:33	29:41	29:51	30:03
28:40	28:55	29:02	29:09	29:12	29:22	29:29	29:38	29:43	29:51	30:02	30:13
28:50	29:05	29:12	29:19	29:22	29:33	29:40	29:48	29:53	30:02	30:12	30:24
29:00	29:15	29:22	29:29	29:33	29:43	29:50	29:58	30:04	30:12	30:23	30:35
29:10	29:26	29:32	29:39	29:43	29:53	30:00	30:09	30:14	30:23	30:33	30:45
29:20	29:36	29:43	29:50	29:53	30:03	30:10	30:19	30:24	30:33	30:43	30:56
29:30	29:46	29:53	30:00	30:03	30:14	30:21	30:29	30:35	30:43	30:54	31:06
29:40	29:56	30:03	30:10	30:13	30:24	30:31	30:40	30:45	30:54	31:04	31:17

SEA LEVEL 5K-time	FEET ABOVE SEA LEVEL										
	2000	3000	3500	4000	4500	5000	5500	6000	6500	7000	7500
29:50	30:06	30:13	30:20	30:24	30:34	30:41	30:50	30:55	31:04	31:15	31:27
30:00	30:16	30:23	30:30	30:34	30:44	30:52	31:00	31:06	31:15	31:25	31:38
30:10	30:26	30:33	30:40	30:44	30:55	31:02	31:11	31:16	31:25	31:36	31:48
30:20	30:36	30:43	30:51	30:54	31:05	31:12	31:21	31:27	31:36	31:46	31:59
30:30	30:46	30:54	31:01	31:04	31:15	31:22	31:31	31:37	31:46	31:57	32:09
30:40	30:56	31:04	31:11	31:15	31:25	31:33	31:42	31:47	31:56	32:07	32:20
30:50	31:06	31:14	31:21	31:25	31:36	31:43	31:52	31:58	32:07	32:18	32:31
31:00	31:17	31:24	31:31	31:35	31:46	31:53	32:02	32:08	32:17	32:28	32:41
31:10	31:27	31:34	31:41	31:45	31:56	32:04	32:13	32:18	32:28	32:39	32:52
31:20	31:37	31:44	31:52	31:55	32:06	32:14	32:23	32:29	32:38	32:49	33:02
31:30	31:47	31:54	32:02	32:05	32:17	32:24	32:33	32:39	32:48	33:00	33:13
31:40	31:57	32:04	32:12	32:16	32:27	32:34	32:44	32:49	32:59	33:10	33:23
31:50	32:07	32:15	32:22	32:26	32:37	32:45	32:54	33:00	33:09	33:21	33:34
32:00	32:17	32:25	32:32	32:36	32:47	32:55	33:05	33:10	33:20	33:31	33:44
32:10	32:27	32:35	32:42	32:46	32:58	33:05	33:15	33:21	33:30	33:42	33:55
32:20	32:37	32:45	32:53	32:56	33:08	33:16	33:25	33:31	33:41	33:52	34:05
32:30	32:47	32:55	33:03	33:07	33:18	33:26	33:36	33:41	33:51	34:02	34:16
32:40	32:57	33:05	33:13	33:17	33:28	33:36	33:46	33:52	34:01	34:13	34:27
32:50	33:08	33:15	33:23	33:27	33:39	33:46	33:56	34:02	34:12	34:23	34:37
33:00	33:18	33:25	33:33	33:37	33:49	33:57	34:07	34:12	34:22	34:34	34:48
33:10	33:28	33:36	33:43	33:47	33:59	34:07	34:17	34:23	34:33	34:44	34:58
33:20	33:38	33:46	33:54	33:58	34:09	34:17	34:27	34:33	34:43	34:55	35:09
33:30	33:48	33:56	34:04	34:08	34:20	34:28	34:38	34:43	34:53	35:05	35:19
33:40	33:58	34:06	34:14	34:18	34:30	34:38	34:48	34:54	35:04	35:16	35:30
33:50	34:08	34:16	34:24	34:28	34:40	34:48	34:58	35:04	35:14	35:26	35:40
34:00	34:18	34:26	34:34	34:38	34:50	34:58	35:09	35:15	35:25	35:37	35:51
34:10	34:28	34:36	34:44	34:48	35:01	35:09	35:19	35:25	35:35	35:47	36:01
34:20	34:38	34:46	34:55	34:59	35:11	35:19	35:29	35:35	35:45	35:58	36:12
34:30	34:48	34:57	35:05	35:09	35:21	35:29	35:40	35:46	35:56	36:08	36:23
34:40	34:58	35:07	35:15	35:19	35:31	35:40	35:50	35:56	36:06	36:19	36:33
34:50	35:09	35:17	35:25	35:29	35:42	35:50	36:00	36:06	36:17	36:29	36:44
35:00	35:19	35:27	35:35	35:39	35:52	36:00	36:11	36:17	36:27	36:40	36:54

SEA LEVEL	FEET ABOVE SEA LEVEL										
5K-time	2000	3000	3500	4000	4500	5000	5500	6000	6500	7000	7500
35:10	35:29	35:37	35:45	35:50	36:02	36:10	36:21	36:27	36:38	36:50	37:05
35:20	35:39	35:47	35;56	36:00	36:12	36:21	36:31	36:38	36:48	37:01	37:15
35:30	35:49	35:57	36:06	36:10	36:23	36:31	36:42	36:48	36:58	37:11	37:26
35:40	35:59	36:07	36:16	36:20	36:33	36:41	36:52	36:58	37:09	37:22	37:36
35:50	36:09	36:18	36:26	36:30	36:43	36:52	37:02	37:09	37:19	37:32	37:47
36:00	36:19	36:28	36;36	36:41	36:53	37:02	37:13	37:19	37:30	37:42	37:57
36:10	36:29	36:38	36:46	36:51	37:04	37:12	37:23	37:29	37:40	37:53	38:08
36:20	36:39	36:48	36:57	37:01	37:14	37:22	37:33	37:40	37:50	38:03	38:18
36:30	36:49	36:58	37:07	37:11	37:24	37:33	37:44	37:50	38:01	38:14	38:29
36:40	37:00	37:08	37:17	37:21	37:34	37:43	37:54	38:00	38:11	38:24	38:40
36:50	37:10	37:18	37:27	37:31	37:45	37:53	38:04	38:11	38:22	38:35	38:50
37:00	37:20	37:29	37:37	37:42	37:55	38:04	38:15	38:21	38:32	38:45	39:01
37:10	37:30	37:39	37:47	37:52	38:05	38:14	38:25	38:32	38:43	38:56	39:11
37:20	37:40	37:49	37:58	38:02	38:15	38:24	38:35	38:42	38:53	39:06	39:22
37:30	37:50	37:59	38:08	38:12	38:26	38:34	38:46	38:52	39:03	39:17	39:32
37:40	38:00	38:09	38:18	38:22	38:36	38:45	38:56	39:03	39:14	39:27	39:43
37:50	38:10	38:19	38:28	38:33	38:46	38:55	39:06	39:13	39:24	39:38	39:53
38:00	38:20	38:29	38:38	38:43	38:56	39:05	39:17	39:23	39:35	39:48	40:04
38:10	38:30	38:39	38:48	38:53	39:07	39:16	39:27	39:34	39:45	39:59	40:14
38:20	38:40	38:50	38:59	39:03	39:17	39:26	39:37	39:44	39:55	40:09	40:25
38:30	38:51	39:00	39:09	39:13	39:27	39:36	39:48	39:54	40:06	40:20	40:36
38:40	39:01	39:10	39:19	39:24	39:37	39:46	39:58	40:05	40:16	40:30	40:46
38:50	39:11	39:20	39:29	39:34	39:48	39:57	40:08	40:15	40:27	40:41	40:57
39:00	39:21	39:30	39:39	39:44	39:58	40:07	40:19	40:26	40:37	40:51	41:07
39:10	39:31	39:40	39:49	39:54	40:08	40:17	40:29	40:36	40:48	41:01	41:18
39:20	39:41	39:50	40:00	40:04	40:18	40:28	40:39	40:46	40:58	41:12	41:28
39:30	39:51	40:00	40:10	40:14	40:29	40:38	40:50	40:57	41:08	41:22	41:39
39:40	40:01	40:11	40:20	40:25	40:39	40:48	41:00	41:07	41:19	41:33	41:49
39:50	40:11	40:21	40:30	40:35	40:49	40:58	41:10	41:17	41:29	41:43	42:00
40:00	40:21	40:31	40:40	40:45	40:59	41:09	41:21	41:28	41:40	41:54	42:10

Here is how you can use Table 10.1 to determine a realistic race finish goal if you are going from low elevation to high elevation to race, or if you are traveling from a high elevation locale to run a race at a lower elevation.

How to Determine a Race Time Going from Low to High

- Go to Table 10.1 and find your recent 5K race time or an estimated 5K time.

- Next, find the elevation of your race across the top of the table and go to the cell at the intersection of your race time in the elevation column.

- If the race you are doing at altitude is a 5K, then you have your target race time.

- If the race is a 10K, a half-marathon, or a marathon, you can go to Table 3.1 and use your altitude-adjusted 5K time to find the predicted adjusted goal race time.

For example, your recent 5K time at sea level is 24:00, but you are planning a trip to Denver to run a half-marathon. Using Table 3.1, your 24:00 predicts a half-marathon time of 1:51:14. Using Table 10.1 above, your altitude-adjusted 5K time for 24:00 at 5,280 feet is 24:44. Using Table 3.1, your altitude-adjusted equivalent performance half-marathon time is now 1:54:40. That gives you a realistic goal for your half-marathon in Denver.

How to Determine a Race Time Going from High to Low

- Go to Table 10.1 and find the elevation of the city of your race across the top of the table.

- Next, go down the column to find your 5K race time or an estimated 5K time at your high-elevation-city race.

- Look across the row to the left to find the 5K time that corresponds to the column with the lower elevation of the race you intend to run.

- If the race you are doing at altitude is a 5K, then you have your target race time.

- If the race is a 10K, a half-marathon, or a marathon, you can go to Table 3.1 and use your 5K-adjusted time for the lower elevation to find the predicted adjusted goal race time.

In that way, the altitude-adjusted table can also be used by the runner in Denver who is traveling to a sea-level race to set a race goal. The runner in Denver whose 5K time is 24:44 could use Table 10.1 to find the equivalent sea-level time of 24:00. Using a similar procedure as in the previous paragraph, the 24:44 5K time that predicts a 1:54:40 half-marathon for the Denver runner now becomes a predicted half-marathon race time of 1:51:14, based on the sea-level-adjusted 5K time of 24:00.

||||||

REAL RUNNER REPORT

Hi Bill,

I have just finished my second half-marathon using your FIRST training plan, and wow what an improvement! Two years ago, I completed a rather hilly half in 2 hours 4 minutes, using a five-runs-per-week training plan. I never felt fully recovered and my joints began aching from all the "junk miles."

This time around, I followed your plan (albeit without the cross-training) and, despite having two weeks off training just before the race, due to a nasty throat infection, I finished another equally hilly half-marathon in 1 hour 56. My training had been much faster than that, but I was happy with it, given my break from training, and it proved to me that the training works!

I have now read your book and now that I understand the science behind it, I will be able to engage with it even more robustly! I am looking forward to using your marathon plan for my first marathon in April 2018. I am definitely going to be doing the cross-training and strength exercises this time around after reading the book and can't wait to see the results!

Many thanks,
Dani Plowman
NHS Project Manager
West Sussex, UK

AN UPDATE: ————————————————————————————

Hi Bill,

I ran my first marathon in 3:52, which I am super happy with.

Running Injuries

The American Academy of Physical Medicine and Rehabilitation estimates that 70% of runners will become injured at some point in their running career. It is common for FIRST to receive messages from runners describing a recent injury and asking what to do about their training for an upcoming race. I don't hesitate, based on my experiences both as a runner and a coach, to urge runners to stop running and get an evaluation of the injury from a health professional, preferably a physical therapist or an orthopedist who is familiar with running-injury treatment. Treating soreness or injury symptoms early diminishes the length of recovery and the time missed from running. Early intervention can also reduce the likelihood of an injury becoming serious.

Unfortunately, runners are often in denial about an injury or, if they do recognize it, they hope that they can simply "run through it." Sometimes you can, but that's rare. Continuing to train with an irritation usually worsens the inflammation. More than one runner has written me, stating that she is nearing the end of a long preparation for an important race and that "taking time off now is not an option." More likely than not, she will write me several weeks later, saying that she can no longer run and that it hurts even to walk.

At some point during their running lives, most runners will have to face a decision of whether to continue training or to stop and heal.

Like many runners, I have suffered miserably with plantar fasciitis and Achilles tendonitis because I kept training through the soreness and pain. Both injuries are devilishly difficult to recover from, especially when you continue training after detecting the symptoms. The more inflamed the tissue, the longer the recovery. Now I take preventive and rehabilitative measures at the first hint of an irritation. With an appropriate training program and a conservative approach to irritations, downtime from running can be kept to a minimum.

Pay close attention to your body and keep your body in good shape. Think about what a physical therapist or chiropractor would include in your injury rehabilitation—stretches and strength training to address poor flexibility and muscular weaknesses. We advocate doing stretches and strength training as *prehab* rather than *rehab*. The flexibility and strength training exercises and the form drills that we have included in this book can be done in a reasonable amount of time and not only will improve performance, but will provide a good defense against injury.

Many runners have reported that reducing the number of days and miles they run has worked to address their injuries. By eliminating the injuries, these runners are able to train with the intensity needed to improve their fitness and running performance. It is gratifying that the FIRST program is enabling runners to pursue and achieve running goals that, because of previous injuries, they thought were no longer attainable.

We have found it difficult to convince runners to reduce their running as soon as they incur an irritation, regardless of the statistical evidence we can present. When runners contact us about an injury and we ask how long they have been having problems, the answer is often "months." We insist that the runners we coach inform us as soon as they recognize any symptom of injury. We immediately have them reduce their distance and pace. If that doesn't help to relieve the problem, we reduce the frequency of running. We also suggest other conservative treatments, along with the reduced training. By insisting that these guidelines be followed, we have been able to help runners continue their training with only minor modifications, rather than a significant training interruption.

Below we answer commonly asked questions about injuries and describe in some detail the most common running injuries, the causes, the signs and symptoms, and the treatments.

Running Injuries: Q & A

Q. *What are acute injuries?*

A. Strains, partial tears of muscle, sprains, and partial tears of ligaments and tendons usually occur as a result of a fall, a twisting movement, or a forceful, explosive movement, and are classified as acute injuries. The immediate application of compression, ice, and elevation of the injured area will reduce the inflammation and swelling. Seek medical help if the pain or swelling is severe. Rest the affected part until the pain and swelling are greatly reduced or absent. Begin a return to activity by strengthening the injured area, followed by a gradual return to full activity.

An injury does not necessarily preclude activity altogether. You may be able to bike or swim, depending on the specific location of the injury.

Q. *What are overuse injuries?*

A. Overuse injuries are chronic orthopedic irritations, resulting from repetitive strain on a body part. Running contributes to repetitive stress on muscles, tendons, and bones. Without adequate recovery, overuse injuries can develop. The body can recover from most of this stress, but only if it has adequate time for the tissue to adapt, compensate, and grow stronger. Just how fast the adaptation occurs is related to the runner's age, overall physical condition, and the gradual progression of increased training.

Q. *How much running is too much?*

A. This question has no easy answer. There is a wide range among individuals as to their tolerance for running frequency and duration. Frequency and duration of running are two of the factors that determine the overall stress. Adding days of running must be balanced against the increased likelihood of injury. The length of runs must be gradually increased. Too much, too often leads to injury.

Q. *Is training intensity associated with injuries?*

A. Intense training is a fundamental part of the FIRST approach. Intensity brings the greatest gains in performance, while at the same time presenting the opportunity for injury. How to balance increasing intensity with preventing overuse injuries is one of the challenges that all runners face. The intensity (pace) must be gradually increased. Yet just because you are capable of running faster doesn't mean that you should be doing so in each workout.

Increased intensity, or running faster, for your workout should not be done while also increasing distance. Manipulate only one of the three primary training variables—frequency, duration, and intensity—at a time. Increasing more than one variable at a time significantly increases your risk of incurring an injury. However, once an overuse injury has been suffered, the primary treatment will be to reduce intensity.

In particular, be careful with track repeats if you are not accustomed to that type of intense training. Running fast provides many cardiorespiratory benefits, but it also changes running form and, for some, that can mean transferring the stress to a different set of muscles.

Q. *How can overuse injuries be prevented?*

A. To prevent overuse injuries, the runner needs a prudent, well-defined program of running. The design of FIRST's three-days-a-week program is ideal for runners who may be injury-prone. With the appropriate intensity and mileage determined for each workout, the runner can attain improved running performance while reducing the risk of injury. Elite runners who are willing to bear the risks of injury associated with greater intensity, frequency, and duration of effort are not likely to find our approach appealing. For the average competitive runner, however, the costs of pushing to the limits, as measured in injuries and lost training days, are not likely to be worth the marginal improvements.

Q. *How do I know if I have a biomechanical or anatomical problem?*

A. These two categories are not mutually exclusive, and one can lead to the other. A specialist may need to examine both your stride and the biomechanical structure of the lower half of your body. Gait analysis, using high-speed video or digital techniques, is effective, but it can be costly. Talk to your sports medicine physician about what is available in your area. There may be a clinic for runners that can assist you in this endeavor.

At the FIRST Running Retreats, held on the Furman University campus, a gait analysis is performed on each runner. All the retreat participants receive videos of their running, with accompanying remarks about their running form. In addition, they are given recommended stretches and strength-training exercises to perform to address any weaknesses identified in their running.

Q. *What about non-steroidal anti-inflammatory medicine in treating/ preventing running injuries?*

A. Non-steroidal anti-inflammatory (NSAID) medications are very useful in reducing the inflammation associated with different types of running injuries. Their use is often indicated during the recovery from overuse injuries, but they should not be used to permit training by masking the inflammation. You should treat these as medicine, and not as performance boosters. Doing so may lead to greater injury and other complications. Consult with your physician before using NSAIDs.

Q. *Do I need orthotics?*

A. Orthotics are inserts placed in the shoe to correct certain biomechanical problems, such as overpronation or flat feet. Orthotics may be helpful to a runner with bad alignment who is suffering from pain and repeated injuries. A sports medicine doctor can evaluate whether orthotics would be beneficial.

Q. *How does excess body weight affect running injuries?*

A. Body weight has a big impact on running performance and injuries. Carrying too much body weight reduces performance and puts significant additional strain on the joints, ligaments, and muscles. At our FIRST Running Retreats, we find that most runners are disciplined when it comes to their training, but they often lack discipline when it comes to their food choices and consumption. Two problems result from their poor dietary habits—being malnourished and overweight—which compromise optimal training and racing.

The Most Common Running Injuries

We asked physical therapist Dr. Phil Gregory to identify the most common running injuries he treats in the Furman Sports Medicine Center. Phil lectures and performs gait analyses at the FIRST Adult Running Retreats. He is not only an experienced runner, but he has analyzed and treated many runners. Here, he provides a description of each common running injury, its symptoms, and the recommended treatments.

Runner's Knee

"Runner's knee" (RK) is a bit of an umbrella term indicating pain around or behind the kneecap. RK often presents as an irritation around the front of the knee. In addition to pain with running, there may be pain with movements such as squatting and climbing stairs, or stiffness following prolonged sitting. Occasionally, there may be swelling around the kneecap. RK often develops because of overuse. The tissues around the front of the knee may become irritated when there is an increase of activity that exceeds the tissues' ability to adapt and recover.

Other contributing factors include weakness of the muscles of the hip and quadriceps, muscles that help to control and stabilize the bending of the knee. Additionally, increased tightness of the quadriceps and hamstring muscles, or excessive flexibility of the foot, may contribute to increased stress on the knee.

Like most running-related injuries, RK is what is called a "self-limiting condition." That means that activity and training can be continued as tolerated, but they must be reduced to some degree to allow for the tissues to recover. The approach to treatment also depends on effectively identifying the underlying cause. In cases of simple overuse, training must be modified and decreased to allow for proper recovery.

Changes to your running gait may also be beneficial. Specifically, increasing your cadence by up to 5% will help to decrease the load that is placed on the kneecap during running. Other modifications to your stride include landing with the foot underneath your hips, and making sure the kneecap keeps pointing forward, rather than collapsing inward, during the stride. It can be helpful to have a friend video you from the side and from behind to make sure the foot lands underneath your hips and the knee is not rotating inward. Improving strength of the quadriceps and hip muscles is important in more effectively dispersing and absorbing the impact of the running stride.

Treatment

- Increase your running cadence by 5%.

- Improve specific flexibility through stretching exercises: kneeling hip flexor stretch, standing calf stretch, hamstring stretch.

- Foam-roll to improve your range of motion in the quadriceps, iliotibial band, and calves.

- Strengthen the quadriceps, but find a method that is pain-free for you:
    o Single-leg squats
    o Box step-ups
    o Leg presses

- Other strength training:
    o Clamshell
    o Single-leg bridge
    o Lateral step with mini-band

Iliotibial Band Syndrome

The "iliotibial band" (ITB) is a thick band of connective tissue that runs from the muscles on the side of the hips and pelvis, down the side of the thigh, and attaches to parts of the side of the knee. Some fibers of the ITB attach to the side of the kneecap, while other parts of it attach to the outside of the lower leg. The role of the ITB is to help stabilize the pelvis and thigh when standing on one leg (such as during the running stride). With ITB syndrome, there is a feeling of sharp or burning pain on the side of the knee. Typically, this begins to occur at a certain distance into a run and worsens as the run continues. Eventually, it may become painful when performing daily activities, such as going up and down stairs.

One often-overlooked contributor to this condition is running on a road with a sloped shoulder. The tilt of the road can place increased stress on the ITB and the side of the knee. Also, overpronation can result in stress on the ITB as well. The increased motion of the foot during overpronation leads to increased strain on the ITB as it tries to stabilize the leg as it rotates inward. Weak gluteal muscles are a likely risk factor for ITB syndrome, as the gluteal muscles attach to the ITB and help in controlling the inward rotation of the leg during the running stride.

Treatment

- While the iliotibial band cannot be stretched, it may be helpful to improve the overall flexibility around the hips by doing stretches such as the kneeling hip flexor stretch, the piriformis stretch, and the pigeon pose stretch.

- Effective strengthening exercises for this condition include lateral walk with mini-band, hamstring curl with stability ball, single-leg bridge, and clamshell exercises.

Achilles Tendinopathy

The Achilles tendon (AT) is a springlike tissue that connects the muscles of the lower leg to the foot, helping to generate a powerful push off the ground. Clinicians have begun to use the term *tendinopathy*, as pain often develops in the AT without any actual inflammation. Irritation in the tendon occurs because of overuse or biomechanical issues. Because of the role the muscles of the lower leg play in the running stride, the AT can often see loads of two times body weight or more during each step. Unfortunately, this is a very common injury for runners, and up to 50% of all runners will experience this injury during their career.

With Achilles tendinopathy, pain is located at the back of the heel, and can be provoked by squeezing or pinching the tendon. There may be swelling present at the back of the heel or an increased thickening of the tendon itself. Oftentimes, symptoms of stiffness in the ankle may occur following a period of inactivity, such as after sleep or prolonged sitting. Symptoms often improve as the tissue warms up, but may worsen with fatigue, such as at the end of a run.

Risk factors that may contribute to the development of this condition include changes in training, such as a rapid increase in volume, increased speed work, or increased hill work. Changes to footwear, such as switching to a shoe that has a lower heel-to-toe drop, may also place increased stress on the AT. Additionally, tightness in the muscles of the calf can lead to increased tension on the AT, and weakness of those calf muscles can cause the AT to have more strain placed on it during the running stride. Increased pronation of the foot places increased stress on the AT as it helps to stabilize the foot.

Treatment

- The use of a heel lift can help to decrease strain on the AT and alleviate pain.

- Switching to shoes with a higher heel-to-toe offset may also help to decrease strain on the AT.

- Foam-rolling of the calf muscles may also alleviate the symptoms associated with Achilles tendinopathy. It may also be helpful to stretch the muscles of the hip, with exercises such as the kneeling hip flexor stretch and the pigeon pose.

- Exercises to strengthen the calf are the most valuable tool for recovering from Achilles tendinopathy. Standing and seated calf raises help to strengthen the different muscles that attach to the AT and should be done in a progressive way based on your symptoms. When the AT is highly irritated, it can be helpful to only do a few slow reps standing on both feet. As symptoms improve, it's helpful to progress to single-leg calf raises with an increasing number of reps.

- General limb strengthening with exercises such as single-leg squats, single-leg dead lifts, and lateral walks with mini-band can also help to strengthen the larger muscles of the leg to better stabilize the foot and decrease strain on the AT.

Plantar Fasciitis

While *plantar fasciitis* (PF) may be a funny phrase to say, it is certainly not a funny injury to deal with. PF is also the most common foot injury that is seen in the clinic. The plantar fascia is a band of connective tissue that attaches from the base of the heel and extends to the toes. The band acts as a support structure for the arch of the foot, helping to create stability of the foot and control pronation. Injury develops when this tissue becomes stressed beyond its ability to recuperate. This presents as pain and tenderness to the touch at the bottom inside of the heel. One of the classic signs of PF is pain at the heel when first putting the foot on the ground after getting out of bed in the morning.

Common contributing factors to the development of PF include limited range of motion at the big toe and ankle joints, tightness of the muscles of the calf and hamstring, weakness in the muscles of the foot and lower leg, and excessive standing and weight-bearing activity (whether through increasing running volume too quickly or employment that involves extensive standing and walking).

Treatment

- Cushioned shoes, heel pads, and orthotics can help make walking around and standing more comfortable throughout the day.

- Over-the-counter inserts are just as effective at relieving pain as expensive custom inserts. While there are many different styles and brands of inserts, a device that has arch support and a cushioned heel will be most effective.

- The standing calf stretch variations (knee straight and knee bent) help to improve flexibility throughout the foot and decrease strain on the plantar fascia.

- Massage can also help to stretch the fascia. Rolling the foot over a small ball or using your thumbs to dig into the soft tissue of the arch can help to loosen the tissue around the bottom of the foot and decrease strain on the plantar fascia.

- While sometimes uncomfortable to sleep with, a night splint can help to improve the flexibility of the foot and plantar fascia and help with recovery.

Stress Fractures

Stress fractures are often one of the more frustrating injuries for runners, as they often seem to come from nowhere, and the only thing that truly heals them is time. Just as every other tissue adapts to training, bone also goes through changes as part of the training process. The accumulation of impact from the running stride causes bone to go through a cycle of breakdown and growth. With proper recovery, bones become stronger and more robust. With excess training and not enough rest, however, bone can gradually weaken, causing stress fractures.

Runners commonly get stress fractures in the long bones of their feet, along the lower portion of their shin, or even in the bones of the thigh and pelvis. Additionally, nutrition can play an important role in the development or prevention of stress fractures. Runners who do not absorb enough calcium, or those who have conditions such as osteopenia or osteoporosis, may be at increased risk. Women, especially those who often miss their menses, tend to be at higher risk than men. Additionally, those runners who drink excessive amounts of diet soda, specifically dark sodas, may be at increased risk.

Stress fractures are typically associated with very specific, localized tenderness and soreness. Swelling may also be noted at the fracture site, especially with stress fractures of the foot and lower leg. While some injuries feel better once you warm up and get moving, the pain of a stress fracture often continues to increase as you continue running.

Treatment

- Rest is the primary treatment for stress fractures. Typically, four to eight weeks of no running will resolve the problem, but it's equally important to slowly return to training.

- For fractures of the foot and lower leg, a walking boot may be prescribed by your physician to promote healing.

- Cross-training can help to maintain fitness, but activities that involve minimal weight bearing, such as swimming, deep water running, or bicycling, should be emphasized.

- Changes to your running form may be helpful. Specifically, trying to land quietly or softly has been shown to decrease impact.

- When the stress fractures are fully healed, drills such as barefoot strides (faster-paced running for four to six reps of approximately 60 yards) on the grass can help teach you to land more softly during your stride.

||||||

REAL RUNNER REPORT

Bill and Scott,

I want to thank you so much for taking my running to the next level. I qualified for the Abbott Age Group Marathon World Championships, which will take place within the 2020 London Marathon, by following your plans and guidance. I have been a recreational runner since high school, culminating with my first marathon in New York City in 1997 (4:23:30), when I was 34. I took some years off to have kids, and once the youngest was in preschool, I laced up my running shoes again.

I found that running was even more important to me than before, because it restored my body back to pre-pregnancy fitness and it was the best stress relief. I had officially caught the marathon bug, and over the ensuing eight years, I ran 14 marathons, including five Bostons, with a PR at the California International Marathon 2018 of 3:26:48.

In 2016 I joined the Impala Racing Team, an elite all-women's racing team in San Francisco. Running had become such a big part of my life, I wanted to be sure to take all necessary steps to staying injury-free and healthy so I could maintain running as long as possible. I read every running book I could get my hands on, and then I read *Train Smart, Run Forever*.

I thought the science and philosophy behind the book were spot-on, and I signed up for the FIRST Running Retreat in May 2019. The retreat was transformative, and I understood at a deep level what I needed to do to take my running further: I needed to train smarter by making all my runs quality runs by adding intensity, and using cross-training, strength training, and stretching as a regular part of my routine.

I identified the Berlin Marathon 2019 as my fall focus race, and I carefully followed the FIRST plan that Bill gave me. I had never pushed myself that hard during the long runs and tempos, nor had I ever done five 20-milers during a training cycle. I found myself getting faster and stronger. At the Berlin Marathon, where I earned my Abbott World Majors Six Star, at age 56, I achieved a PR with a 3:23:53 and came in 10th in my age group.

I then received the wonderful news that because of my strong marathon times in 2019, I was invited to compete in the Abbott Age Group Marathon World Championships. I am training for it right now, using your FIRST training plan, and I am aiming for another PR. I can't thank you enough for encouraging me to push myself harder to see what I truly can accomplish, while giving me the tools to stay injury free and strong.

Best,
Gina Edwards
Former Attorney
President of the Impala Racing Team
San Francisco, California

12

Running Nutrition

When runners contact FIRST, asking for assistance with their running, they are asked to list an area of their running that needs improvement. Most also cite a need to improve dietary habits. Before attending a running workshop, participants complete a three-day dietary journal. We analyze their food consumption and provide detailed information about their macro- and micronutrients, as well as their daily caloric intake. What we observe is that runners, like most Americans, fail to eat a balanced diet that is composed primarily of fruits, vegetables, and whole grains. It is not uncommon for runners to report a disproportionate number of calories derived from alcohol.

Runners who train vigorously and assiduously often are not as willing to be as disciplined with their eating. We are convinced that they fail to reach their performance potential because they are swayed by misleading information, do not understand how nutrition affects performance, and are not properly fueled for their training. We have seen runners in our training studies improve dramatically as a result of improved nutrition, just as much as they improve from dedicated and smart training. Most of the runners attending our lectures and participating in our training studies indicate that they are confused about dietary guidelines or they have difficulty adhering to them. That's certainly understandable because nutrition is a complex topic. Unfortunately, the avalanche of books touting unsound dietary regimens has not made it easier for runners to be well-informed about proper nutrition.

This chapter does not provide a comprehensive look at nutrition. Over the last 40 years, sport and exercise scientists have conducted numerous nutritional studies in an effort to determine how to best enhance human performance through food and drink consumption. In this chapter, the focus is on fueling the body for performance, both in training and in racing.

Nutrition: Q & A

Q. *Does the training diet for a runner differ from that of the general population?*

A. In general, it does not. A nutritious and healthy dietary plan is based on a selection of fruits, vegetables, and whole grains that have complex carbohydrates as a major component. The runner's diet differs from the general population's in its need for additional fluids to cover sweat losses and additional energy to fuel physical activity. Much of that additional energy should be supplied by complex carbohydrates. By selecting primarily unrefined carbohydrate products, runners also decrease their risk of contracting several chronic diseases, including diabetes, heart disease, and cancer.

Q. *Why should I consume so many carbohydrates?*

A. Keep in mind that when exercising at a low intensity (~30% of aerobic capacity), the fuel used by muscles is mainly from stored fat; at 40–60% intensity, fats and carbohydrates are used evenly by muscles; at 75% intensity, carbohydrates are mainly used by muscles for energy; and at 85% intensity, muscles rely exclusively on carbohydrates. You can see why runners, whose training is almost always at 70% and greater intensity, need to have a readily available store of carbohydrates in the muscles. The contributions of fat and carbohydrates during exercise change with intensity; this is commonly referred to as the "crossover concept" and the point where the contribution of fat shifts with carbohydrates is influenced by the amount and intensity of exercise.

Carbohydrates supply the immediate energy needs of the body and are the major source for glycogen, which is the stored form of carbohydrates in the body. A high-carbohydrate diet ensures the runner a full glycogen load for training and competition.

Minimizing the consumption of simple sugars will help a runner avoid a roller-coaster effect in blood glucose levels. Adding fruits as a dessert choice is a healthier option than refined-sugar desserts. Fruits, like other unrefined carbohydrates, add lots of important vitamins and minerals, and, in some cases, fiber.

Intense training requires that carbohydrates be replaced daily. Since the FIRST training approach is based on high-quality running, it is important that your daily diet be based predominantly on complex (that is, unrefined) carbohydrates.

Q. *Will consuming more protein increase my running performance?*

A. Protein does not provide a significant amount of energy when you run or work out. Protein is the major building material of the body and is essential for tissue growth and repair. A diet based on 15–20% protein will meet both of these needs. The body cannot store protein; any extra is stored as fat, with little being used for your immediate energy needs.

Q. *How much fluid does a runner need to consume prior to training and racing?*

A. Hydration needs are affected by environmental conditions, intensity, duration, body size, fitness, acclimatization, altitude, and genetics. Because of all those variables, it is difficult to prescribe precise levels of fluid consumption. In particular, sweat rates vary from runner to runner and with weather conditions.

It is important to stay adequately hydrated. Two hours before a workout, drink 16 ounces of your preferred sports drink or water. Two hours is ample time for the fluid to be cleared from the stomach and for the kidneys to remove the excess. Hyperhydration increases the risk of a runner's need to urinate during training and racing, with no performance advantage over normal hydration.

In general, thirst is a reliable protective mechanism for determining your hydration needs.

You need to practice drinking during your training, both to train your body to handle fluids during exercise and to learn while working out what is a comfortable amount for you to drink. The longer the event, the more important it is to follow a predetermined hydration schedule, especially when fluid loss from sweating is exceeding the ability of your system to process added fluids.

Q. *How much fluid consumption do you need during exercise?*

A. During exercise the goal is to prevent a significant water deficit. Fluids with sodium and potassium help replace sweat losses. Sodium stimulates thirst and fluid retention, and carbohydrates provide energy. Beverages containing 6–8% carbohydrates are recommended for events longer than 60 to 90 minutes. Consuming eight ounces every 30 to 40 minutes, depending on thirst, is adequate under normal climatic conditions. Most runners prefer cool, flavored beverages.

Q. *What fluid is best to drink while training for a race?*

A. Well before race day, contact the event promoters to find out what types of fluid replacement will be available or out on the racecourse. During your long runs, practice with the race-day drink to get used to it. You do not want to find out on race day that your stomach can't handle the event drink.

Q. *Can I drink too much water?*

A. Yes, especially during prolonged exercise. For the last several years, runners have heard the mantra "Hydrate, hydrate, hydrate." Hydration is good and important, but during long runs some runners drink too much fluid. This results in a dilution of the body's sodium stores, leading to hyponatremia. Hyponatremia is a potentially dangerous state and can be a life-threatening condition; in fact, hyponatremia has been responsible for several marathoners' deaths over the past years. Use your weight loss during exercise as a guide for fluid replacement.

The popularity of the marathon has resulted in the participation of runners with a vast range of talent. Marathon times have increased to an average of over four hours, with many runners still on the road five to six hours after the start. Many of these runners have trained with groups that stress the importance of fluid intake throughout the course of the race. Due to the low workload related to their pace, these runners actually gain water weight as a result of consuming more water than they have lost by sweating. This results in lower sodium concentrations in their blood and has the potential to lead to hyponatremia. Because the symptoms may resemble those of dehydration, hyponatremia victims are often given liquids, only worsening their condition.

Q. *How should I determine my post-workout and -race fluid replacement?*

A. Weigh yourself before a race or a long run and then weigh yourself afterward; during the rest of the day, consume 16 ounces of fluid for every pound lost.

Q. *What should I eat before racing?*

A. Eating before exercise, as opposed to fasting, has been shown to improve performance. General guidelines include consuming food relatively low in fat and fiber, high in carbohydrates, moderate in protein, and, importantly, foods familiar to the runner. The size and timing of meals are interrelated.

Individuals must determine the type and quantity of food to eat before a race, as well as when they will consume the meal. To work out your personal plan, begin with the information below and, through trial and error on long-distance training days, vary the type, quantity, and timing of meals. Maintain an accurate log of these variables and your long-run performances to determine your most effective and agreeable pre-race meal plan.

For a simple way of estimating your caloric needs on race morning, use this formula:

(Hours before race)	X	(body weight in pounds)	=	(number of calories to consume)
(Hours before race)	X	(body weight in kilograms x 2.2)	=	(number of calories to consume)

For example, if you wake up at 6:00 a.m. and your race is at 8:00 a.m., that's two hours. So, for a 150-pound runner, that's 2 x 150 = 300 calories. Four hours before the event, a 120-pound runner would consume 480 calories; a 150-pound runner 600 calories.

Typically, consuming 300 to 500 calories three hours before a half-marathon or a marathon, followed by 100–150 calories of sports drink an hour prior to the race, should supply adequate pre-race fuel.

For shorter races lasting less than an hour (5K and 10K), fewer, if any, pre-race calories are necessary.

Your pre-race plan should not include any new food or drink. Your experimentation with what best fuels your long runs adequately without causing GI issues should occur during your training. You've heard the phrase "Nothing new on race day"; this applies to nutrition and hydration as well. Your pre-race fueling should be routine by the time of the race.

Individuals vary widely in how much food and drink they need and in what concentrations they can tolerate. Your experimentation is more important than what any textbook recommends.

Common pre-marathon fueling foods include oatmeal, bananas, bagels, toast, peanut butter, and sport bars. Some runners prefer to consume mostly liquid calories. I have found that an eight-ounce can of a meal supplement (such as Ensure or Boost) provides 220 calories and 32 grams of carbohydrates. If you are worried about too much bulk in the stomach, the meal supplement can give you 440 calories with only 16 ounces of liquid. The calorie-dense supplemental meal does not inhibit gastric emptying, so you won't have a heavy feeling in your stomach.

I prefer eating three to four hours before a marathon. I want to make sure I have consumed enough calories to be prepared for the multihour event. I also want to make sure that I have eaten early enough to ensure elimination, so I won't need to interrupt my race for a pit stop.

Q. *What should I consume during exercise?*

A. In general, for races and workouts that are less than 60 to 90 minutes, your pre-run caloric intake and hydration should be adequate, and nothing will be needed during your activity. For races and workouts longer than 90 minutes, the American College of Sports Medicine recommends that you consume 30 to 60 grams, or 120 to 240 calories, of carbohydrate every hour. If you drink eight ounces of 6% sports drink, which provides 14 grams of carbohydrate, every 20 minutes, you will consume 42 grams per hour, or 168 calories. Depending on temperature, humidity, and individual sweat rate, consuming eight ounces every 30 minutes may be adequate, which still provides 28 grams of carbohydrate, or 112 calories. Depending on the race distance, that may be sufficient.

Some runners like to use energy gels during marathons. Consuming an energy gel with water every hour can also help maintain adequate blood glucose levels.

Whatever your preference is for consuming calories during a long endurance event, whether that is gels, sports drinks, or food, it is important for you to have practiced that consumption regimen during practice. Remember: Nothing new on race day.

Q. *Do I need special nutrition for competition? How about carbohydrate loading?*

A. Exercise increases the energy requirements of the body up to 25 times those of normal expenditure. The body converts all carbohydrates to glucose, which may be used immediately as fuel or stored for later use. Glycogen is the stored form of glucose in the body, mostly in the skeletal muscles and liver. The body has a limited storage capacity for glycogen, which may be rapidly depleted during strenuous exercise.

During exercise that feels easy, over half the calories used for energy are from stored body fat. As exercise intensity increases to moderate, the body begins to burn less fat and utilize more glycogen—that is, stored carbohydrates. Long runs tend to deplete glycogen. The term "hitting the wall" is used to describe the effect that glycogen depletion has on a runner.

Once your stored glycogen is depleted, your body shifts back to burning fat. Because converting fat to energy cannot be done as efficiently as using glycogen for energy, your pace decreases.

One aim of training is to increase the pace at which you can run while burning fat. In other words, your easy pace becomes a faster pace. By burning fat, rather than glycogen, you put off glycogen depletion; that is, you put off hitting the wall. Appropriate training increases the pace you can maintain before your crossover from fat burning to carbohydrate burning occurs, helping to save glycogen that will be needed further down the road.

If you maintain a diet that is high in complex carbohydrates, it is not necessary to carbohydrate-load. As you begin a taper, your activity level will decline; thus you will burn fewer of your carbohydrate stores. Your normal high carbohydrate diet (60–70% of total calories coming from carbohydrates), combined with a decrease in activity (for your taper), will result in carbohydrate-loading. The day before your race, your diet should also be high in carbohydrates, but refined carbohydrates may make a better choice because of their reduced fiber content.

The most efficient energy yield from stored glycogen occurs with an even running pace. A fast pace early in the race speeds the depletion of glycogen and leads to hitting the wall.

Perhaps the only dietary adjustment needed is a slight reduction in total caloric intake during race week, just as the volume of your exercise is reduced prior to a race.

Q. *What should I consume after a workout or race?*
A. The workout or race is over and you are feeling exhausted. Now is the time to start replenishing the glycogen and fluids lost during the effort. Sports drinks are a good option. The body is a carbo-

hydrate sponge immediately after intense and exhausting exercise. Glycogen resynthesis from carbohydrates consumed after exercise takes place most rapidly during the first 30 minutes after exercise. Foods with a high glycemic index that are absorbed quickly into the bloodstream may speed up the replenishment of glycogen in skeletal muscle because they stimulate a rapid rise in glucose and insulin. During the first two hours following exercise, try to take in solid foods that are high in carbohydrates, such as bagels, bananas, pudding, etc. Recommended replacement includes 200–400 calories of carbohydrate and 40–50 calories of protein with sufficient fluid. The timing and composition depend on the duration and intensity of your exercise session and on when your next intense workout will occur. The sooner you refuel, the sooner your muscles will have the tools necessary to recover.

Final Comments

Running, as with all activities carried out by the body, requires energy. Sports nutrition is a complex issue, and this chapter provides basic guidelines for fueling your training and racing. It is not a sports nutrition manual. Only basic nutritional information for your training and racing is provided. For more specific dietary information, FIRST recommends consulting with a sports nutritionist.

REAL RUNNER REPORT

Hi,

I wanted to give you a positive email for a Monday morning. I've followed your RLRF programme over the past three years. I wrote after getting a BQ in my first marathon in 2014. I dropped my PR by 8 minutes in my second marathon in 2015 and ran Boston in 2016, making some tapering and diet mistakes, and running 3 h 45 as a result.

Today I ran the London Marathon in 3 h 14:48 at age 56, using the programme as the basis for some extra runs—I've still struggled with the cross-training. So good for age and guaranteed entry to London, and good for age for New York. I have just bought your new book after hearing you talk on marathon training and going to try to cross-train more.

Two big points for me.

1. I did my last 20-mile run two weeks before and tapered for two weeks, not three.

2. I forced myself to really rest yesterday and to eat 10 grams per kg carbs. No wall, almost even splits between two halves. 1:37:14 & 1:37:34.

Thank you. You are inspiring. As you can tell, I'm very happy this evening. I got the feeling back I had in the first marathon of being strong in the second half.

Andy Mellon
Paediatrician
Newcastle-upon-Tyne, United Kingdom

13

Body Composition

It's the lean and muscular runners who cross the finish line first. That's because body composition and weight significantly influence running performance. Try wearing a 10-pound weighted vest or carrying a couple of 5-pound dumbbells on your next run if you need to be persuaded that a few extra pounds make a difference in your pace. Finding your optimal body weight is similar to the importance of finding the right pace for optimal training for your best running and good health.

Addressing body weight with runners, especially young women, has become a taboo topic. However, it is too significant an issue to ignore. Not only does being too heavy or too thin contribute to less than optimal performance, but it also undermines good health. We are reluctant to talk about weight loss because of the prevalence of eating disorders among runners, both young and old. But finding a healthy body weight that enables vigorous training, coupled with sustainable healthy dietary habits, is important.

For good health, we are most concerned with body composition. Body composition is a measure of body fat and fat-free mass, including bone, muscle, connective tissue, fluid, and organ tissues. Having excess body fat is described as being overweight or obese. Both of these conditions contribute to the onset of diabetes, high blood pressure, some types of cancer, and other major medical problems and diseases. Even physically active, fit runners can be overweight or obese.

An increase in body fat content results in a reduction in aerobic capacity, or VO$_2$ max. As discussed in Chapter 6, maximal oxygen consumption is a major determinant of running performance. Gaining body fat will reduce your fitness level. Similarly, reducing excess body fat will improve your fitness level.

What Is a Healthy Body Composition?

Most people tend to make judgments about their health based on their body weight. Although a scale can provide your weight, it does not assess the composition of your weight. It is excess body fat that poses a health risk. Furthermore, your scale does not show where your fat is stored. Fat stored in the abdominal area poses a significant health risk. Population studies typically use body mass index (BMI) to track weight classifications because computing it only requires you to know your weight and height. It does not differentiate between body fat and fat-free weight. An individual may be overweight by the BMI measure, while being very muscular with a low percentage of body fat. Similarly, an individual may be underweight by the BMI measure, while having a high percentage of body fat. BMI is not a good measure for assessing an individual's body composition, especially for an athlete. At the FIRST lab, we utilize measurements from the most recognized and accurate methods of estimating lean mass. These methods have low error rates.

Table 13.1 presents FIRST body composition standards developed from our experiences with testing runners, as well as healthy body composition recommendations from various health organizations, such as the American College of Sports Medicine, the American Council on Exercise, as well as scientific and epidemiological studies. The table provides categories of body fat percentages, ranging from the athletic runner to what is considered unhealthy and risky. Loss of muscle mass begins by age 30 and becomes increasingly difficult to maintain with aging. That's why resistance training is important throughout a lifetime.

At our FIRST Retreats, we collect body composition measurements on our participants. They are always anxious about the results. Oftentimes, runners are shocked that their body fat percentage is as high as it is. This might be because, compared to the general public, these runners are relatively thin. Given the American rates of obesity and overweight, simple comparisons with the general public are not necessarily good indicators of healthy weights. It is common for runners to think that, because they are disciplined runners, they are healthy. Excess body fat can even jeopardize the health of dedicated runners.

TABLE 13.1

Body Fat Ratings

BODY FAT RATING	FEMALES	MALES
Risky	> 39%	> 30%
Excess Fat (Overfat)	30 – 35%	25 – 29%
Borderline Overfat	29 – 34%	20 – 24%
Lean	23 – 28%	13 – 19%
Competitive	15 – 22%	5 – 12%
Risky	< 15%	< 5%

Compared to the average American's tendency to become overweight or obese with aging, are runners who engage in vigorous physical activity three times per week or more able to maintain a "healthy weight" as they age?

A survey was conducted of 297 runners from 40 states and 12 countries who attended one of FIRST's running workshops between 2007 and 2018. Because the runners who attend the running workshops devote four days and several thousand dollars (travel, lodging, etc.) to further their knowledge about running and training, it is reasonable to describe them as dedicated and committed runners.

These recreational runners with an average age of 50 years, who attended one of the workshops, were chosen for the study to see how successful they had been years later in pursuit of their goal of lifelong running and what changes in training and health they had incurred.[1] The study surveyed workshop participants to examine their running frequency, injuries, body weight changes, and supplemental training as they aged.

Oftentimes, runners report that they run so they can eat what they want. They commonly report that they run to manage their weight. At the workshops, runners have their body composition assessed. In general, runners are dedicated and disciplined. They train year-round in all types of weather and devote considerable time to their sport. They are aware that running performance is influenced by body weight. They also report that their running goals are of great importance to them. In most cases, all that is holding them back is their excess body weight.

The survey results from this study illustrate the positive influence running has on weight management for these dedicated runners. Compared to the percentage of the general public who are obese (39.8%), the 6.1% obesity rate of the dedicated runners is a strong testament to the value of running as a healthy behavior.[2] Similarly, comparisons of those respondents with healthy weights to the general public are another endorsement of running as a beneficial physical activity. On the other hand, the 31% rate of male survey respondents classified as overweight is perplexing, given their goals and dedication to physical activity.[3] Only 13% of the female runners were overweight years after attending the retreat. The difficulty that even dedicated runners have in maintaining healthy and performance-enhancing body weight illustrates the challenge presented by the cultural and environmental influences that contribute to excessive caloric intake.

REAL RUNNER REPORT

Hi Team,

I write to give you some positive feedback on your efforts and say a big thank-you for your FIRST program.

I used the program as a guide to training for my first marathon and was more than happy with the result. Three hours 7 minutes, and finishing fast (42nd km was my fastest), was an extremely satisfying outcome for a first attempt, the Melbourne Marathon (Australia), by a 56-year-old man.

I work as a tradesman and spend plenty of time on my feet, so I was attracted to a low kilometer program. I have been a recreational runner for a couple of years and a firm believer in quality and effort, over miles and hours. As such, I was attracted to the FIRST program, as it is a perfect fit for my philosophical approach to training.

It is fair to say that many of the people I run with were extremely dubious of my methodology. Every time I told a seasoned veteran that I would only complete a single training run over 30km before the big day, they would look at me like I was naive, at best, or more commonly, a fool, who was going to get what he deserved on the big day. Now the results are in and my time bettered every person I run with over a range of age groups from their 20s to me. It seems FIRST and I are entirely vindicated.

I did make a couple of adjustments to the program. Although I was prepared to believe that by following the long-run program I would be physically capable of covering the 42km, I wanted to be mentally confident, so I tweaked the long run. I stretched it to 35km, and punched out the last 5km in PMP [planned marathon pace]. On the same principle of building confidence, I attacked the 21km and recorded a time (1:27) that convinced me I was on track.

So, thanks again. I am over the moon with my result and grateful for your efforts. Keep up the good work.

Kind Regards,
Peter Rushen
Painter
Melbourne, Victoria, Australia

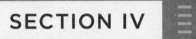

SECTION IV

ESSENTIAL ELEMENTS TO BE A FIT FIRST RUNNER

14

Strength Training for Runners

Nowhere is the adage "Use it or lose it" more relevant than when it comes to muscles. Running tends to employ one set of muscles over and over, while neglecting others. Runners must also combat the loss of muscle mass that is a natural part of the aging process. It is imperative that we do strength exercises as we age to diminish the loss of muscle tissue.

Most adults lose about half a percent of their muscle mass each year after the age of 25.[1] This loss accelerates after the age of 60. Muscle mass is associated with metabolism. Muscle activity increases caloric expenditure. Strength training builds muscle and bolsters metabolism—a key to maintaining your desired weight.

If you wish to be fit, fast, and healthy, you must include strength training in your regular exercise routine. We are aware that many runners do not. It is evident from their posture and their inability to do resistance exercises. Maintaining muscle mass is important for reducing injury risk, for enhancing physical performance, for maintaining or improving body composition, and for maintaining overall good health. As we age, balance, agility, and coordination are diminished through the loss of muscle mass.

A strong musculature can better absorb the stressful impact on the body from repetitive foot strikes. Without adequate muscle mass for the absorption, bones and connective tissue suffer. Stress fractures are much more common among thin runners. The more the muscles absorb the shock, the less the bones need to do so. Strengthening the calf will help to reduce the stress on the ankle and tibia. Strengthening the quadriceps and hamstrings will reduce the stress on the femur.

Running speed is determined by stride length and stride frequency. Stride length is increased if there is more power available in the push-off phase of the gait. Having more power comes from being stronger in the hips and lower extremities. Resistance training will help to develop the muscle strength that provides more power during the push-off phase of the running cycle.

Type II, or fast-twitch, muscle fibers tend to be reduced in number and size with aging sooner than slow-twitch fibers.[2] Strength training can help to retain fast-twitch fibers, which can contribute to a runner's ability to run fast. We all want to be able to sprint to the finish line.

Fat-free mass is a major determinant of VO_2 max. Resistance training contributes to producing more fat-free mass. Runners can raise their fitness level by increasing their fat-free mass. Too many runners are worried about nothing but total body weight. They need to be more concerned about their body composition.

Runners attending our retreats are surprised by how difficult it is for them to perform some of our strength exercises. That's because they have neglected to do functional strength training. Functional strength training involves performing resistance exercises specific to the movements of your sport.

Regardless of your strength-training schedule, consistency is the key. Weight training, resistance training, strength training—they are all the same. Since this chapter focuses on training that will work the musculoskeletal system and will frequently use body weight as the resistance, the term *strength*, rather than *weight* or *resistance, training* is used predominantly. There is no consensus regarding the optimal scheduling of strength training for runners.

For the enhancement of your running, we have described strength-training exercises that can be performed in a relatively short period and will contribute to better running and injury prevention. In Chapter 16, "Putting It All Together with the 7-Hour Workout Week," we have a schedule for how you can fit strength training into your weekly workouts.

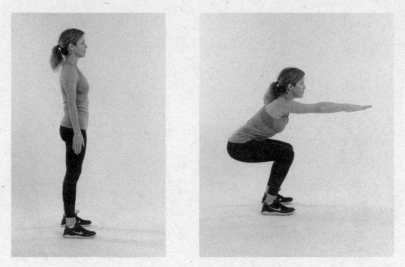

BODY-WEIGHT SQUAT

- Stand with your feet hip-width apart and your arms down by your sides.

- Keeping your back straight, your core tight, and your knees pointing in the same direction as your feet, squat down, bending at your hips and knees until your thighs are parallel to the floor.

- Keep your weight on your heels, rather than on the front of your feet, so that your knees do not extend beyond your toes.

- Place your hands on your hips or extend your arms out in front to help maintain your balance.

- In a controlled movement, return to the starting position by extending the knees and hips until you are standing in an upright position.

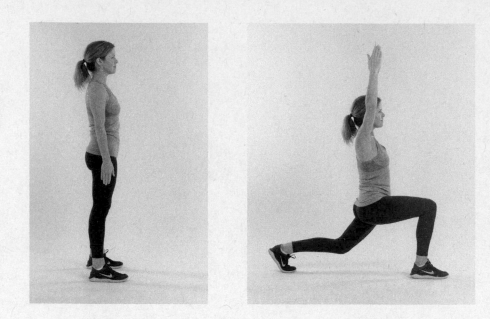

WALKING LUNGES WITH HANDS OVERHEAD

- Begin standing with your feet hip-width apart and your arms by your sides.

- Maintaining an upright posture, raise your arms overhead and take a step forward with your right leg, landing on your right heel as you bend your knees in a forward lunge.

- Your front thigh should be parallel to the floor. Keep your back knee from touching the ground.

- Both knees should bend, and the front thigh should be parallel to the floor.

- Avoid stepping so far forward that your front knee extends beyond the point of your front toes. Your lead knee should point in the same direction as your foot throughout the lunge.

- Push off with your forward foot to bring your back leg forward, stepping into a lunge on your left side.

- Continue stepping forward, alternating legs the prescribed number of reps for each leg (see Chapter 16).

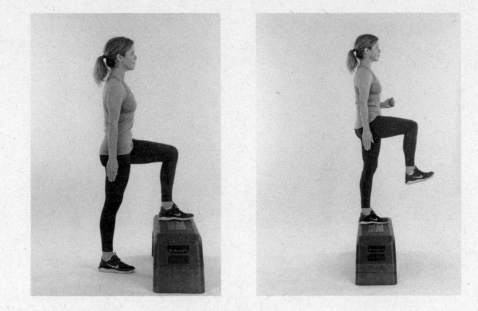

BOX STEP-UPS

- Find a sturdy box with a height so that when your foot is on top of the box, your thigh is parallel to the ground.

- Use your left leg to raise yourself up by extending your left hip and knee to stand up on top of the box.

- Use your left leg to lift the rest of your body up and try to avoid pushing up with your right foot.

- Step down with the right leg and return to the original standing position. Repeat with the left leg for the prescribed repetitions (see Chapter 16), then switch to the right leg for the required repetitions.

- Keep your torso upright during the box step-ups. Your forward knee should point in the same direction as your foot.

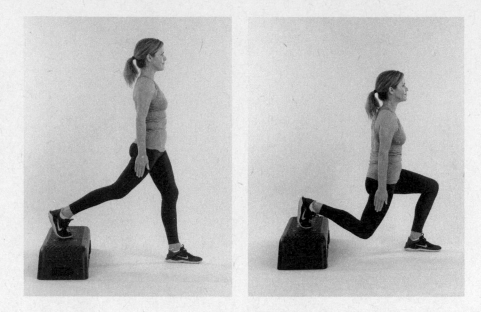

ELEVATED SINGLE-LEG SPLIT SQUAT

- Stand in front of a knee-high bench with your feet hip-width apart and your hands by your side.

- With your right foot on the bench, step forward with your left foot (about 18–20 inches in front of the bench).

- Keeping your torso upright and your hips facing forward, squat down by flexing your left knee and hip until your left thigh is almost horizontal and until your right knee is almost in contact with the floor.

- Be careful to keep your left knee in line with your left foot and do not allow your left knee to travel beyond your left foot.

- Drive up through your left heel back to the upright starting position. Avoid pushing through the right (elevated) leg.

- Repeat and continue with equal reps on the opposite leg.

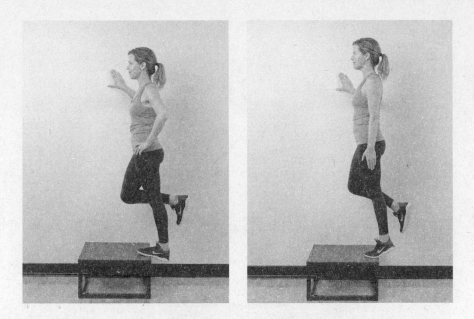

SINGLE-LEG CALF RAISE

- Stand on an elevated surface (e.g., a step, a box, or a curb) with your feet hip-width apart.

- Position the balls of your feet with the heels and arches of the foot extending off the surface.

- Place a hand on the wall or a support for balance.

- Lift your right leg behind you by bending your right knee.

- Lower your left heel by bending at your ankle until your calf is stretched.

- Lift up with your left heel by extending your ankle as high as possible.

- Pause briefly then lower back to the starting position.

- Keep your left knee straight throughout exercise.

- Repeat and continue with equal reps on the opposite leg.

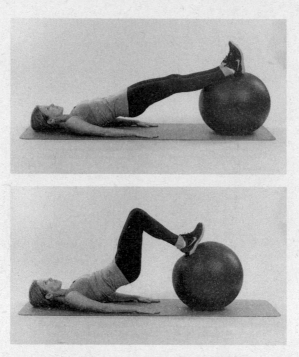

HIP-EXTENSION LEG CURL WITH EXERCISE BALL

- Lie on your back on the floor, with your feet on top of an exercise ball and your arms by your sides.

- Position the ball so that when your legs are straight, your ankles are on top of the ball.

- Raise your hips off the ground, keeping your weight on your shoulder blades and your feet until your body forms a straight line from shoulders to heels. This is your starting position.

- Keep your hips high and pull your heels and the exercise ball toward your butt as close as you can.

- Keep your glutes tight and avoid dropping your butt toward the ground.

- Keeping your hips high, let the ball roll back slowly as you straighten your legs and return to the starting position.

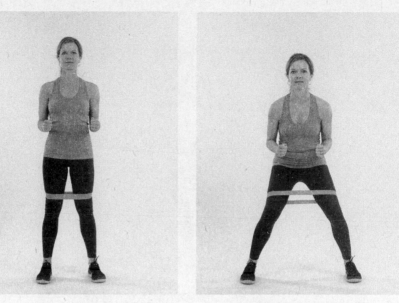

LATERAL STEP WITH MINI-BAND

- Place a mini-band above your knees (you can lower the mini-band toward your ankles as you improve your strength).

- Stand with your feet hip-width apart to create tension on the band. Maintain an upright posture and look straight ahead. Your toes should be facing forward and your feet parallel.

- Stand with your knees slightly bent and step laterally with one foot and then bring the other leg inward to a new ready position, maintaining tension on the resistance band.

- Step to the right for the prescribed number of repetitions, then step to the left for the prescribed number of steps (see Chapter 16).

- Always keep tension on the band when you are stepping and do not let your feet come together. Keep your feet pointed straight forward during the entire exercise.

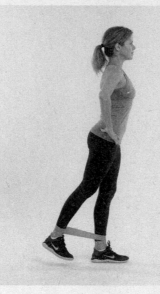

KICKBACKS WITH MINI-BAND

- Place a mini-band just above your ankles.

- Face a wall or use a chair to keep upright and maintain your balance.

- Slightly bend your left leg while you lift the right foot just off the ground. Keep your right leg straight and drive your right foot back behind you.

- Keep your body upright throughout the movement and avoid leaning forward in order to get the leg farther up behind you.

- With a controlled motion, pause at the back of the leg swing and then return to the starting position. Repeat on the same side for the prescribed number of repetitions (see Chapter 16), then switch sides.

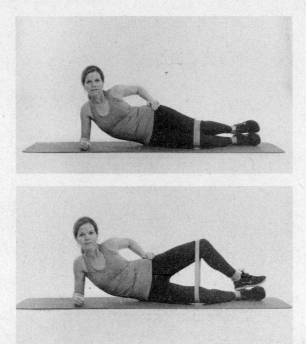

CLAMSHELL WITH MINI-BAND

- Place a mini-band around your legs just above your knees.

- Lie on your right side, propped up on your forearm, with your left leg stacked on top of your right leg and your knees bent at a 45-degree angle. Your heels should be in line with your butt.

- Raise your top knee toward the ceiling as high as you can. Keep your feet together and avoid rotating your pelvis or back. Your lower leg remains on the floor during the exercise.

- Hold for a second at the top, then slowly lower your knee to the starting position.

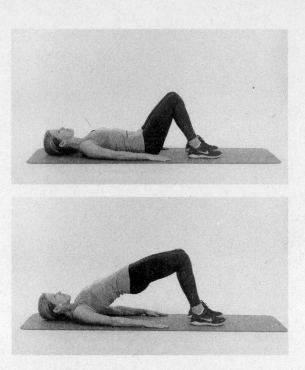

BRIDGE/PELVIC THRUST WITH FEET FLAT

- Lie on your back with your feet flat on the floor.

- Place your arms at your sides, with the palms on the floor next to your hips.

- Pressing into the floor with your hands and feet, exhale as you tighten the hamstring and gluteal muscles and lift your pelvis upward to form a straight line from shoulders to knees.

- Make sure you are driving straight up and your knees stay apart.

- Pause for one second, then slowly lower the hips toward the ground, but not all the way.

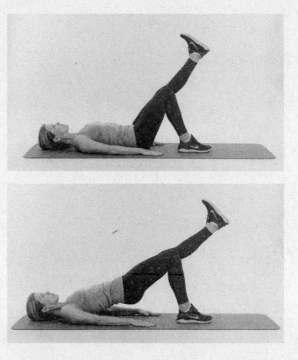

SINGLE-LEG BRIDGE/PELVIC THRUST

- Lie on your back with your feet flat on the floor.

- Place your arms at your sides, with the palms on the floor next to your hips.

- Straighten your left leg and hold it even with the right leg.

- Keeping your right foot flat on the ground, press into the floor with your hands and feet, exhale, and lift your pelvis upward to form a straight line from shoulders to knee.

- Make sure you are driving straight up and your knees stay apart.

- Pause for one second, then slowly lower your hips toward the ground, but not all the way.

- Repeat the exercise with the opposite leg.

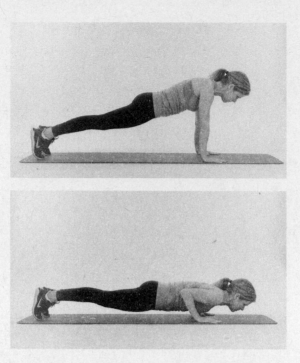

PUSH-UPS (STANDARD OR MODIFIED)

- Get into a high plank position with your hands on the ground, directly under your shoulders. Brace your core (tighten your abs), keeping your back straight.

- Lower your body, keeping your back straight until your chest grazes the floor. Do not let your hips sag or point up.

- Your body should remain in a straight line from head to toe.

- Keeping your body straight, exhale as you push back up to the starting position.

- Keep your hips straight throughout the entire movement.

MODIFIED: Perform the exercise with the knees on the floor, keeping your hips straight.

MORE ADVANCED: Perform the push-ups on a BOSU ball.

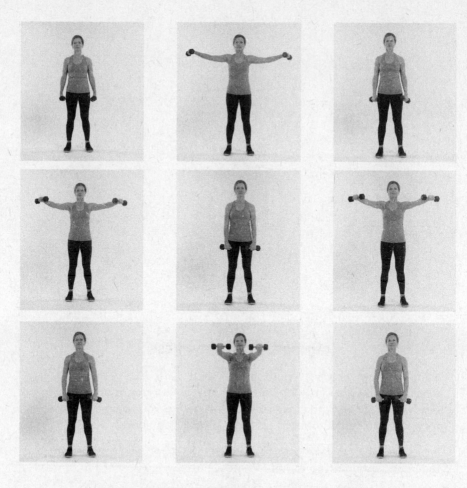

DUMBBELL CLOCKER SHOULDER RAISE

- Visualize the body as the center of a clock and you are facing 12 o'clock.

- Stand, holding a pair of dumbbells by your side, and raise your arms to the 3 o'clock and 9 o'clock positions until your arms are just slightly above horizontal. Then lower.

- Raise your arms to the 2 o'clock and 10 o'clock positions, then lower.

- Raise your arms to the 1 o'clock and 11 o'clock positions, then lower.

- Raise your arms straight in front of you, then lower.

- Repeat this sequence four more times.

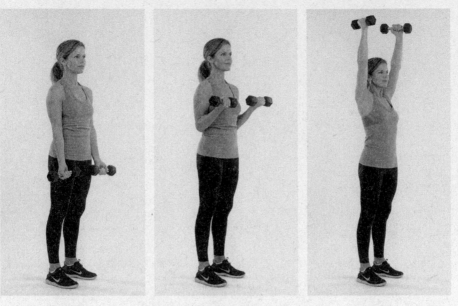

DUMBBELL CURL TO PRESS

- Stand straight, holding a dumbbell in each hand with your arms extended down and by your sides. Keeping your upper arms and elbows stationary and close to your torso with your palms facing forward, curl the dumbbells up toward your shoulders.

- Press the weights over your head, rotating as you go so your palms face each other at the top of the movement.

- Avoid arching your back as you press the weight overhead.

- Lower both arms with control and return your arms to the curl position, then lower to the starting position.

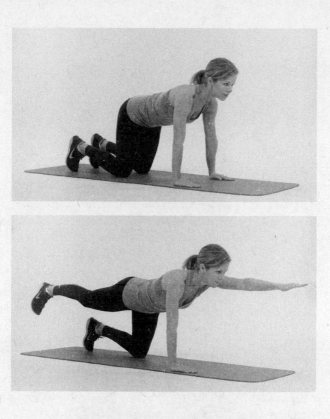

QUADRUPED/POINTER DOG

- On a mat, start on all fours with your hands under your shoulders and your knees under your hips. Your head, neck, and back should be straight.

- During the exercise, keep your head level—not raised upward, in a neutral position—to minimize pressure on your neck.

- Raise your left arm and reach it forward until it is in line with your torso.

- As you bring your left arm forward, straighten and lift your right leg until it is straight and in line with your torso. Hold this position for three seconds.

- Slowly bring your left arm and right leg back to the ground and repeat with the right arm and left leg.

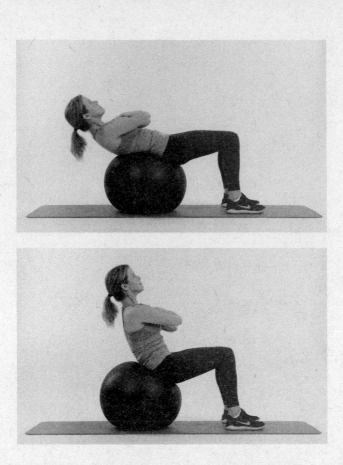

ABDOMINAL CRUNCH ON EXERCISE BALL

- Sit on an exercise ball and place your feet flat on the floor, hip-width apart. Roll back until your lower back is resting comfortably on the ball. Position your arms across your chest, with your hands near your shoulders. Raise your head even with your torso, looking straight up.

- Contract your abs and slowly curl your torso forward to raise your chest up to an upright or vertical position. Raise your chest until you feel your abs completely contract; pause for one second and lower your head and torso back down to the starting position.

- Perform the crunches in a controlled manner and avoid bouncing on the ball; focus on your abs while doing the exercise.

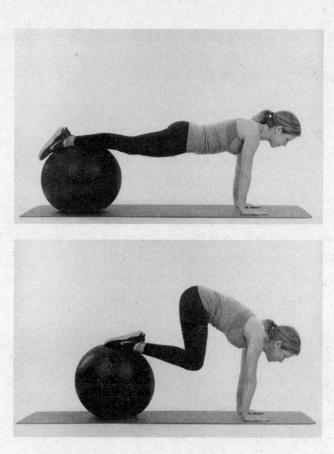

REVERSE CRUNCH WITH EXERCISE BALL

- Lie on an exercise ball on your stomach, with your feet touching the floor behind the ball.

- Lean forward until you touch the floor with your hands.

- Walk your hands away from the ball until you feel the ball reach your lower legs.

- Keep your shoulders directly above your hands. Keep your hands in place, and use your abdominal muscles to roll the ball forward by bending your knees and hips.

- Hold this position for a second and roll back out.

REAL RUNNER REPORT

Good morning, Dr. Pierce and Dr. Murr!

Sorry—long email coming! My name is Natalie Waller, and I am a 40-year-old health and physical education teacher and runner. I first used your plan when training for my first half-marathon back in December 2013; it was the Kiawah Island Half-Marathon, and my goal was just to break 2:00 hours and I did! My time was 1:57:46. It was an AMAZING feeling! I thought that I was going to be one and done with that long of a distance, but here I am almost five years later about to run my 54th half this weekend. lol. I'm working on running a half-marathon in every state.

I have basically been following your plan of three quality runs a week ever since that first half, and I cross-train with swimming, biking, and the indoor rower. I have SWORN up and down that I will NEVER run a full, but the past few months I have been seriously considering it. I've even thrown in a couple of super long runs—16 and 18 miles—recently, just to see how I would feel doing it, and I think I'm going to give it a try. The race I have targeted is on March 2; it's the Snickers Marathon in Albany, Georgia (it's pretty flat). I would LOVE to finish just under four hours, but I'm just not sure which training paces I should follow.

Anyway, I've looked at the training paces for the Key Runs, based on a 23:00 5K, and I don't feel that I can hit them. In my most recent 400s workout, my intervals were 1:43–1:47 and in my most recent 800s workout, my intervals were 3:32–3:40. In the super long runs I did of 16 and 18 miles, my pace was 9:16 and 9:31, respectively. So my question is: Do I base my training paces on the 23:00 5K (equivalent to a 3:43 full, which I feel 100% sure I could never do) or my average half time, which I would say would be close to 1:52/1:53 (equivalent to 3:55/3:58 full time, which is closer to my goal and what I feel is realistic for my ability)? I also realize that the weather on race day will play a huge role; if it's too warm, then I know I won't have a shot to break 4, but I still want to train to try to do it.

Again, I apologize for the super long email! I have really enjoyed following your program and it has helped me to get faster since that first half. I would really value and appreciate any feedback you can give me!

Natalie Waller
Teacher
Fayetteville, Georgia

AN UPDATE

So I took Bill's advice and based my training on the 24:00 5K paces and times. And then I also followed Scott's advice and blended the two marathon training programs since I already had a half-marathon base. I did three total 20-mile runs (actually I did a 20-, a 21-, and a 22-miler). I went in feeling like it was physically possible for me to break 4, based on my times in training, but I honestly had no idea how my body would respond, since it was my first one, plus the conditions yesterday weren't really ideal and similar to what I'd been training in (even though the race was in the same state I live in!). The temps were in the 60s with 90% humidity and minimal wind; it was overcast, though. My strategy was to try to hang with the 3:55 pacer until at least mile 18, and then slow down the pace for the last 8.2. I made it to 20 miles in just under 3 hours, which I was very happy about, so I knew I just had to run an "easy" 10K and I would make it. Well, those last 6 miles were the hardest thing I've ever done—temps were approaching 70 and I was hurting so bad, but I just blasted my "final miles" playlist and kept plodding along and thinking about how amazing it would feel to finish. I'm happy to report that I finished in 3:59:04!! It was the greatest feeling in the world! I'm still in disbelief over it. lol.

Thank you both so much for developing this program and for your feedback and advice when I was starting out. This will definitely not be my last one!

15

Flexibility and Form

Scientific studies may not definitively confirm that stretching helps to prevent injuries. However, what is the first test that a physical therapist, chiropractor, or orthopedist performs on an injured runner? Yes, an assessment of flexibility. Similarly, the first step in rehabilitation is stretching. Just as we explained that we recommend strength training as "prehab," rather than waiting until rehab, the same is true for stretching.

Maybe there are not strong data to support a specific recommendation, but it is well recognized by sports scientists and athletes that flexibility is important for athletic performance. In particular for runners, flexibility of ankles, hamstrings, and hip flexors affects form and performance. A lack of flexibility often leads to strained muscles or connective tissue. We definitely have found that running form and flexibility affect performance. Proper form will improve efficiency and thus, economy. Good form also helps you avoid injuries.

Flexibility is determined by the range of motion across a joint or multiple joints. It is influenced by age, gender, genetics, injuries, activity level, temperature, and time of day. Joint range of motion and muscle flexibility are foundations of functional performance. The American College of Sports Medicine includes flexibility as a component of fitness.

The risk factors associated with poor flexibility include faulty posture, altered running mechanics, impaired running economy, and risk of injury and pain. At our FIRST Retreats we commonly see poor posture among runners with poor flexibility. That poor posture contributes to poor running form, which in turn contributes to inefficiency.

Running economy is the energy cost of running at a specific speed. Poor posture or form causes a runner to expend more energy to maintain a given pace. That causes the runner to be less economical. Using more oxygen and glycogen because of poor mechanics means that the runner is not fulfilling his potential.

A common problem among runners is restricted ankle flexibility. This lack of ankle range of motion (especially the inability to pull toes toward the shin) results in lower extremity injuries—calves, knees, hamstrings, hips—by transferring stress and impact to these lower-extremity sites. Stretching to improve ankle flexibility should be a part of every runner's workout routine.

Because runners typically lose flexibility as they age, a common characteristic of the older runner is a shortened stride. However, shortened strides are not limited to older runners. Any runner with tight hamstrings and a tight lower back will have a shortened stride, which impairs running economy.

We recommend that runners take time to incorporate dynamic stretches into their warm-up before beginning the FIRST Key Runs. The static stretches can be completed in a short amount of time and with consistency contribute to improved flexibility. In keeping with our approach of developing a program that is realistic, effective, and not very time-consuming, we have provided a schedule in Chapter 16 for how stretches can be incorporated into your weekly workouts. Our experience is that most runners don't have the time to devote to extensive stretching and drilling, as collegiate teams and elite runners do. Those runners often devote several hours a day to training. We strive to assist runners with limited time to attain optimal results. Incorporating the stretches into your weekly workout schedule does not take much time, but the benefits are considerable.

Dynamic Stretches Before Run Workout (~5 minutes)

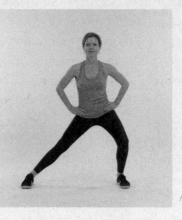

Focus on controlled motion while working toward increasing your available range of motion.

DYNAMIC SIDE LUNGE

- Keeping your feet facing forward, take a wide step out to your left side.

- Let your left hip and knee bend with your body weight over your left foot.

- Keep your right leg straight. Push back up to the starting position and alternate to the other side and repeat.

DYNAMIC SINGLE-LEG DEAD LIFT

- Stand on your left leg with a slight bend in your knee.

- Keeping your spine straight and your right leg straight and in line with your torso, slowly bend forward at the hip and lower your upper body until your torso and right leg are parallel to the floor.

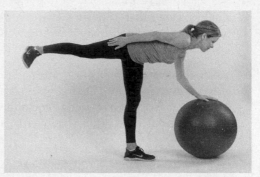

- Return to the upright position and repeat for 30 seconds, then switch to your right leg and repeat for 30 seconds.

DYNAMIC BENT-KNEE FORWARD SWING

- Facing a wall, lean slightly forward at your waist and place your hands on the wall for support.

- With one knee bent at a 90-degree angle, drive this knee up toward your chest to a comfortable height in a rhythmic and controlled motion.

- Gradually increase the range of motion until your leg swings as high as it will comfortably go.

- Repeat with the other leg.

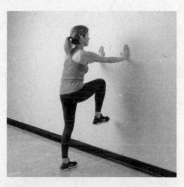

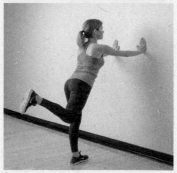

DYNAMIC BENT-KNEE LATERAL SWING

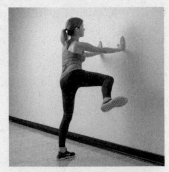

- Facing a wall, lean slightly forward at your waist and place your hands on the wall for support.

- With one knee bent at a 90-degree angle, drive this knee up and across your torso toward the opposite shoulder and then up and out toward the other shoulder.

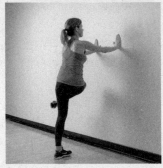

- Gradually increase the range of motion until the leg swings as high as it will comfortably go.

- Repeat with the other leg.

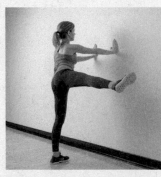

DYNAMIC STRAIGHT-LEG LATERAL SWING

- Facing a wall, lean slightly forward at your waist, and place your hands on the wall for support.

- Keeping your knee straight and leading with your heel, alternate swinging your leg out and away from your body and then across the front of your body in a rhythmical motion.

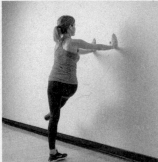

- Gradually increase your range of motion until your leg swings as high as it will comfortably go.

- Repeat with the other leg.

Stretches After Your Run (13–15 minutes)

Try to stretch beyond your available range of motion, but not to the point of pain. Hold each stretch for 30–45 seconds.

OPEN HIGH KNEEL

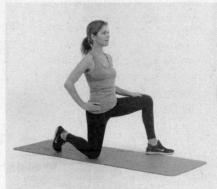

- Kneel on the ground on your right knee, and place your left foot in front of your body.

- Rotate your left leg 90 degrees out to your left side.

- Press your hips forward, keeping your torso straight and your core tight.

- Hold the stretch for 30–45 seconds, then switch sides.

PIGEON POSE

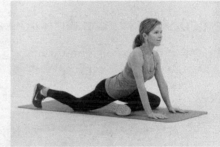

- Place your right leg straight behind you, and your left leg crossed in front of your body.

- Your left shin may angle back toward the right hip or be more parallel to the front of your mat, depending on your flexibility.

- Keep the front of your left leg as flat on the floor as possible.

- Keep your hips square and facing the front of your mat.

- Support your torso with your hands on the ground in front of you.

- Lean your torso forward, keeping your core tight.

- Hold the stretch for 30–45 seconds, then switch sides.

QUADRICEPS STRETCH WITH ROLLER

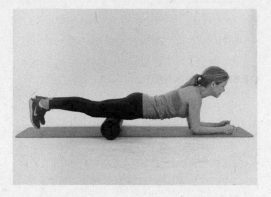

- Lie facedown with a foam roller positioned near your hips, while supporting yourself on your elbows.

- Keep your core tight and your torso straight.

- Using your arms, slowly move your body forward and backward, allowing the foam roller to roll slowly across your thighs.

- You can either do both legs at the same time or one leg at a time. By doing one leg at a time, you can target different angles on the foam roller by turning your feet both in and out.

- Gently roll back and forth for 30–45 seconds.

PIRIFORMIS STRETCH WITH ROLLER

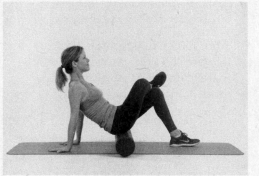

- Sit on a foam roller and place your right ankle on your left knee.

- Lean back slightly with your body weight over your right hip.

- Slowly roll back and forth over the right hip, using your arms and supporting leg to control the pressure to focus on any tender areas.

- Gently roll back and forth for 30–45 seconds, then switch sides.

LOW BACK STRETCH WITH ROLLER

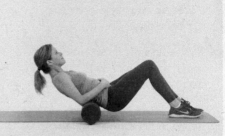

- Lie on the floor with your arms crossed in front of your chest, and a foam roller positioned against your lower back.

- Lift your hips up off the ground, then slowly roll across your lower back.

- Turn slightly to the left and right if there is too much pressure on your spine.

- Gently roll back and forth for 30–45 seconds.

HAMSTRINGS STRETCH WITH ROLLER

- Position a foam roller under your thighs, while using your arms to help hold your hips off the ground.

- Roll back and forth slowly across your hamstrings, focusing on any tender areas.

- Roll with your feet turned in and out to cover the entire muscle group.

- For a more advanced stretch, stack your legs so as to increase the weight on the bottom leg, then switch sides.

- Gently roll back and forth for 30–45 seconds.

ITB STRETCH WITH ROLLER

- Lie on your side, using your forearm to support your upper body.

- Place a foam roller under your mid-thigh, with the foot of the lower leg off the ground.

- Roll slowly along the length of your thigh.

- Keep your opposite foot on the ground for support.

- For a more advanced stretch, stack both legs so there is more weight on the roller.

- Gently roll back and forth for 30–45 seconds, then switch sides.

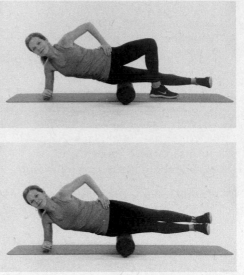

GASTROCNEMIUS STRETCH WITH ROLLER

- Position a foam roller under one calf, while using your arms to support your weight.

- Roll back and forth slowly across the calf.

- Roll from your ankle to just below your knee to target the entire muscle.

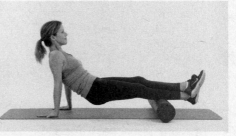

- Gently roll back and forth for 30–45 seconds, then switch sides.

- Focus extra time on tender areas.

Stretches for Cross-Training Days (10 minutes)

Try to stretch beyond your available range of motion but not to the point of pain. Hold stretches for 30–45 seconds.

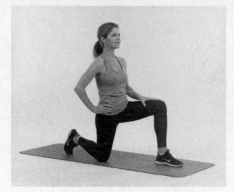
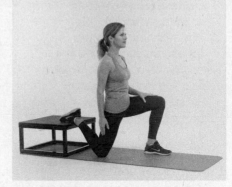

Advanced

TALL KNEELING STRETCH

- Kneel on the ground on your right knee and place your left foot in front of your body.

- Press your hips forward, keeping your torso straight and your core tight.

- Your forward knee should not extend beyond the point of your toes.

- Hold the stretch for 30–45 seconds, then switch sides.

ADVANCED: Elevate the rear foot (e.g., on a box, a bench, or a chair).

HAMSTRINGS STRETCH WITH ROPE

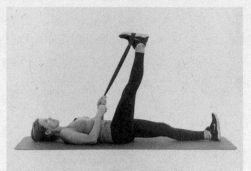

- Lie on the floor on your back, with your legs straight forward.

- Using a rope or a strap around the arch of your right foot, lift your right leg as far as you can toward the ceiling, keeping your knee and leg straight. Use the rope for gentle assistance at the end of the stretch.

- Lower the leg and repeat, trying to lift your leg a little higher.

- For a more advanced hamstring stretch, tighten the hamstrings of the elevated leg to push down into the rope. Resist with your arms while maintaining a static position. Tighten your hamstrings for 10 seconds, then relax and attempt to pull the elevated leg further toward your torso for an additional stretch.

- Hold the stretch for 30–45 seconds, then switch sides.

PIRIFORMIS STRETCH

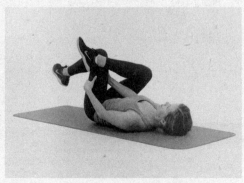

- Lie on the floor on your back, with your knees bent and your feet flat on the floor.

- Bend your right leg and place the ankle in front of your left knee.

- Clasp both hands behind your left thigh and pull your legs toward your torso until a stretch is felt in the right hip and glutes.

- Hold the stretch for 30–45 seconds, then switch sides.

LOW BACK STRETCH #1

- Lie on the floor on your back, with your knees bent and your feet flat on the floor.

- Slowly bring your knees toward your chest and gently grasp your legs below the knee.

- Hold them in place for 30–45 seconds and avoid rocking back and forth.

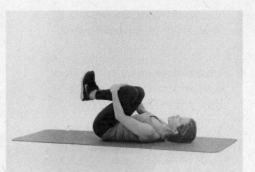

COBRA/PRONE BACK EXTENSION

- Begin in a facedown position on the floor with your palms flat, placed beneath your shoulders.

- Tighten your abs and draw your belly button toward your spine. You want to engage your abs to protect your lower back.

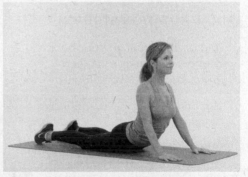

- Spread your fingers and press your palms into the floor.

- Push your upper body off the floor and straighten your arms as much as is comfortable, while keeping your hips, legs, and feet stationary on the floor. Your lower back will be slightly arched.

- Go only as far as is comfortable and stop if you experience any pain. Hold the stretch for 30–45 seconds.

LOW BACK STRETCH #2

- On your hands and knees, drop your hips back toward your heels.

- Lower your chest to the floor and stretch your arms out straight in front of you.

- Hold the stretch for 30–45 seconds.

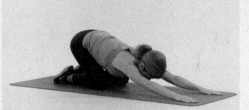

SPINAL ROTATION STRETCH

- Lie on the floor on your back. Bend your knees and keep your feet flat on the floor.

- Extend your arms at shoulder level.

- Slowly let your knees fall toward your left side until you feel a gentle stretch in your back.

- Keep your knees together during the stretch.

- Hold the stretch for 30–45 seconds, then switch sides.

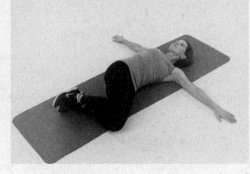

HIP ABDUCTORS/ITB STRETCH WITH SPINAL ROTATION

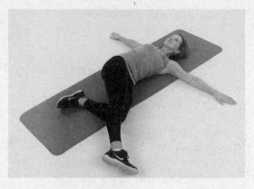

- Lie on the floor on your back. Bend your knees and keep your feet flat on the floor.

- Extend your arms at shoulder level.

- Slowly let your knees fall toward your left side until a gentle stretch is felt in your back.

- Keep your knees together during the stretch.

- Extend the top leg out straight (you can use a rope or a strap to gently pull your straight leg so that it becomes perpendicular to your torso).

- Hold the stretch for 30–45 seconds, then switch sides.

ISOLATED GASTROCNEMIUS STRETCH

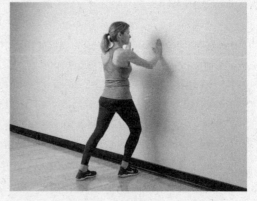

- Facing a wall, place your left leg behind you with the toes of your back foot slightly pointed in.

- Bend your front leg to lean forward against the wall.

- Press your hips toward the wall, while keeping the back leg straight and your heel flat on the floor.

- Hold the stretch for 30–45 seconds, then switch sides.

ISOLATED SOLEUS STRETCH

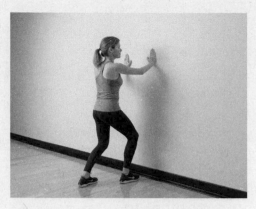

- Facing a wall, place your left leg behind you with the toes of your back foot slightly pointed in.

- Bend your front leg to lean forward against the wall.

- After performing the gastrocnemius stretch, press your hips toward the wall and stretch the soleus by slightly bending the knee of your back leg.

- Maintain this position as you press your hips toward the wall, while keeping your heel flat on the ground.

- Hold the stretch for 30–45 seconds, then switch sides.

|||||| ▬▬▬▬▬▬▬▬▬▬▬▬▬▬▬▬▬▬▬▬▬▬▬▬

REAL RUNNER REPORT

Hi, Scott/Bill,

I just wanted to drop you a quick note to say thank you after completing my first marathon on Sunday.

In 2014 I spent eight days in a coma, fighting for my life battling the effects of an infection, as well as septic shock. Whilst very lucky to come out the other side and eventually fully recover, it was important to me to be able to complete something that I hadn't been able to do prior to being sick. Whilst in the hospital I had adopted the mantra to "Get better not bitter," and running a marathon was a way to prove to myself I was in fact not getting bitter, but better.

I have been a keen runner for many years and competed six half-marathons, but never a full marathon. Whilst recovering from being sick, every time I looked to build out my kilometers I ended up with a soft-tissue injury. I stumbled upon your book and read it cover to cover on a flight from Sydney to London, and you guys had me hooked. And by the time I landed, I had already mapped out a schedule for myself to slowly build up my kms to run the Sydney marathon this year.

I work a relatively busy job and have two small children, so your programme not only gave me the opportunity to build up my kms without the extra stress on my leg muscles, but enabled flexibility in my schedule.

This previous Sunday I completed the Sydney marathon in a time of 3 hours 38 minutes and already am planning my next. It was truly a fantastic experience and I honestly believe that without your programme it's something I would never have been able to experience.

I am very grateful for the programme that you guys developed and I hope you guys are aware of the difference that this has made to my life and a sense of accomplishment I have been able to achieve. I was also able to raise circa $5,000 for the hospital that looked after me whilst I was sick, so hopefully in some way this goes to paying forward the support I have had over the last two years.

Thank you very much and happy running,
Craig Johnston
Banker
Sydney, New South Wales, Australia

16

Putting It All Together with the 7-Hour Workout Week

In our book, *Runner's World Train Smart, Run Forever (TSRF)*, we introduced the 7-Hour Workout Week, based on our experiences as lifelong runners, coaches, and exercise scientists. The 7-Hour Workout Week we are including in this edition of *Run Less Run Faster* differs somewhat from the one in *TSRF*. In *TSRF*, the emphasis was not on getting faster, but on maintaining fitness. We considered it an ideal plan for the runner who occasionally races. The 7-Hour Workout Week presented in this chapter includes FIRST intense aerobic training, focused on improving running performance.

Most runners have busy lives and limited time for training. As we have written throughout this book, we wish to provide a realistic approach with optimal benefits for runners with limited training time. For us, the daily lunch hour is generally our available training period. Seven hours per week, an average of an hour of training each day, will enable you to achieve a high level of physical fitness, be prepared to race, and develop a plan for becoming a lifelong, healthy runner.

The seven hours include activities to enhance cardiorespiratory endurance, muscular strength and endurance, and flexibility. While Scott and I have access to sophisticated training and analytic equipment, we've found that our own training for lifelong fitness is done with minimal equipment—

a stability ball, a stretching mat, a few dumbbells, some stretch bands, and a watch.

Our 7-Hour Workout Week schedule is designed to develop overall fitness and running speed while reducing the likelihood of injury. The schedule was developed with the goal of enabling runners to use it for lifelong running, as well as race preparation for 5Ks, 10Ks, and half-marathons. It is designed for general fitness and health enhancement on a regular basis, even when there is no targeted future race.

The 7-Hour Workout Week is ideal as a base for beginning a marathon training program. We think that with purposeful and focused training, most runners can adequately and appropriately prepare for running races from the 5K to the half-marathon with seven hours of training per week. By extending the length of Key Run #3, as presented in Table 6.5, the program can be used for marathon training. However, when training for a marathon, weekly training time will be increased and may be closer to eight hours a week—still realistic for many runners who are juggling multiple life responsibilities.

Yes, you might become even fitter and maybe even faster by doing more, but you also would risk getting injured and/or burning out, or creating an imbalance with other priorities in your life. This plan is focused on creating a healthy balance among work, family, and other outside interests and pursuits, along with pursuing serious running goals.

The activities included in the 7-Hour Workout Week provide the FIRST Key Runs and the cross-training that are designed for improving cardiorespiratory and running fitness. The plan also includes functional strength training to make you a stronger and more powerful runner and specific stretches to enhance your flexibility for performance enhancement and injury prevention.

Over the past 14 years, since the initial publication of *Run Less Run Faster*, one message from runners is clear: "Just tell me what to do and I will do it." Runners like structure. We have provided a prescriptive workout for each day of the week.

As we developed the 7-Hour Workout Week, we asked ourselves if each workout could be done easily. That is, we wanted to make sure that the workout was not too difficult to perform; that it did not require a specific facility; and that it required minimal equipment. No matter how good an exercise or training plan is, if it isn't something you are likely to do, it will do no good.

We do these exercises ourselves. We know how long it takes to perform them. The benefits from doing the strength exercises, stretches, and cross-training are significant for runners. Many runners have confessed to us that they skip the resistance training, stretching, and cross-training recommended in *Run Less Run Faster*. Yes, runners like to run, just run.

But to become a fit, fast, and healthy lifelong runner requires more than just running. Give the weekly plan a chance to help you become a faster runner. Before we get to the day-by-day plan, here's a brief description of each of the elements.

Run Workouts

The three run workouts included in the 7-Hour Workout Week are the same three Key Runs spotlighted in Chapter 6, "Three Quality Runs." We have documented the success of thousands of runners using those Key Run workouts.

Cross-Training Workouts

The two cross-training workouts included in the 7-Hour Workout Week are the same workouts included in Chapter 7, "Essential Cross-Training."

Strength-Training Exercises

Do the strength exercises designated in the schedule. You can find instructions on how to perform the strength exercises in Chapter 14, "Strength Training for Runners."

Stretches

Do the stretches designated in the schedule. You can find instructions on how to perform the stretches in Chapter 15, "Flexibility and Form."

The 7-Hour Workout Week Summary

Monday	Cross-train 30–40 minutes; strength-train 15 minutes; stretch 10 minutes
Tuesday	Dynamic stretches 5 minutes; run workout of 50 minutes; stretch 10 minutes
Wednesday	Cross-train 30–40 minutes; strength-train 15 minutes; stretch 10 minutes
Thursday	Dynamic stretches 5 minutes; run workout of 50 minutes; stretch 10 minutes
Friday	Strength-train 15 minutes; stretch 10 minutes
Saturday	Dynamic stretches 5 minutes; run 60–90 minutes; stretch 15 minutes.*
Sunday	Cross-train 30 minutes (optional); stretch 10 minutes (or rest day)

* For marathon training, run 90–180 minutes as determined by Key Run #3 distance and pace.

Monday: Cross-Train 30–40 Minutes, Strength-Train 15 Minutes, Stretch 10 Minutes

Choose and complete a cross-training workout from Chapter 7, "Essential Cross-Training."

Strength (Resistance) Exercises (15 minutes)

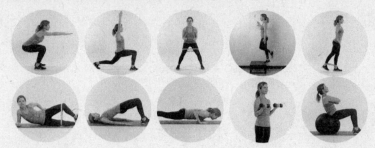

(See Chapter 14, "Strength Training for Runners," for descriptions of the strength exercises.)

Body-Weight Squat
60 seconds

Clamshell with Mini-Band
15 reps each leg

Walking Lunges w/ Hands Overhead
15 steps each leg

Bridge/Pelvic Thrust w/ Feet Flat
20 reps with pause

Lateral Step w/ Mini-Band
15 steps each side

Push-ups (standard or modified)
60 seconds

Single-Leg Calf Raise
15–20 reps each leg

Dumbbell Curl to Press
20 reps

Kickbacks with Miniband
15–20 reps each leg

Abdominal Crunch on Exercise Ball
60 seconds

Stretches (10 minutes)

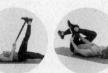

(See Chapter 15, "Flexibility and Form," for descriptions of the stretches.)

Low-Back Stretch #1
30–45 seconds

Tall Kneeling Stretch
30 seconds each side

Cobra/Prone Back Extension
30–45 seconds

Hamstrings Stretch with Rope
30–45 seconds each leg

Low-Back Stretch #2
30–45 seconds

Piriformis Stretch
30–45 seconds each side

Tuesday: Dynamic Stretches 5 Minutes, Run 50 Minutes, Stretch 10 Minutes

---

Dynamic Stretches (Before Run, 5 Minutes)

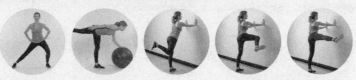

(See Chapter 15, "Flexibility and Form," for a description of the dynamic stretches.)

Dynamic Side Lunge
30 seconds each leg

Dynamic Bent-Knee Lateral Swing
10–15 reps each leg

Dynamic Single-Leg Dead Lift
30 seconds each leg

Dynamic Straight-Leg Lateral Swing
10–15 reps each leg

Dynamic Bent-Knee Forward Swing
10–15 reps each leg

Complete Key Run #1

(See Chapter 6, "Three Quality Runs," for run workouts and target times/paces.)

Stretches (After Run, 10 minutes)

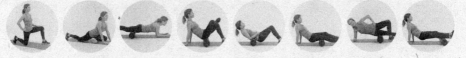

(See Chapter 15, "Flexibility and Form," for a description of the post-run stretches.)

Open High Kneel
30 seconds each leg

Low Back Stretch with Roller
45–60 seconds

Pigeon Pose
30 seconds each leg

Hamstrings Stretch with Roller
30–45 seconds each leg

Quadriceps with Roller
45–60 seconds

ITB Stretch with Roller
30–45 seconds each side

Piriformis Stretch with Roller
45 seconds each side

Gastrocnemius Stretch with Roller
30–35 seconds each leg

Wednesday: Cross-Train 30–40 Minutes, Strength-Train 15 Minutes, Stretch 10 Minutes

Choose and complete a cross-training workout from Chapter 7, "Essential Cross-Training."

Strength (Resistance) Exercises (15 minutes)

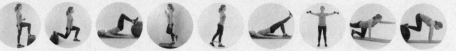

(See Chapter 14, "Strength Training for Runners," for a description of the strength exercises.)

Box Step-Ups
30 seconds up & down w/ right foot; repeat with left foot

Elevated Single-Leg Split Squat
20 reps each leg

Hip-Extension Leg Curl w/ Ball
20 leg curls

Single-Leg Calf Raise
15–20 reps each leg

Kickbacks with Mini-Band
15–20 reps each leg

Single-Leg Bridge/Pelvic Thrust
20 reps each leg with pause

Dumbbell Clocker Shoulder Raise
5 reps at each of the clock positions

Quadruped/Pointer Dog
15 seconds each side w/ pause

Reverse Crunch on Exercise Ball
60 seconds

Stretches (10 minutes)

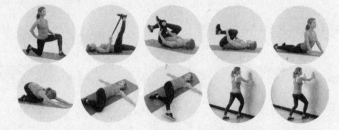

(See Chapter 15, "Flexibility and Form," for a description of the stretches.)

Tall Kneeling Stretch
30 seconds each side

Hamstrings Stretch with Rope
30 seconds each leg

Piriformis Stretch
30 seconds each side

Low Back Stretch #1
30–45 seconds

Cobra/Prone Back Extension
45 seconds

Low Back Stretch #2
30–45 seconds

Spinal Rotation Stretch
30–45 seconds each side

Hip Abductor/ITB Stretch with Spinal Rotation
30–45 seconds each side

Isolated Gastrocnemius Stretch
30 seconds each leg

Isolated Soleus Stretch
30 seconds each leg

Thursday: Dynamic Stretches 5 Minutes, Run 50 Minutes, Stretch 10 Minutes

Dynamic Stretches (Before Run, 5 Minutes)

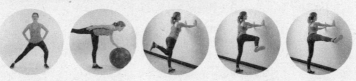

(See Chapter 15, "Flexibility and Form," for a description of the dynamic stretches.)

Dynamic Side Lunge
30 seconds each leg

Dynamic Bent-Knee Lateral Swing
10–15 reps each leg

Dynamic Single-Leg Dead Lift
30 seconds each leg

Dynamic Straight-Leg Lateral Swing
10–15 reps each leg

Dynamic Bent-Knee Forward Swing
10–15 reps each leg

Complete Key Run #2

(See Chapter 6, "Three Quality Runs," for run workouts and target times/paces.)

Stretches (After Run, 10 Minutes)

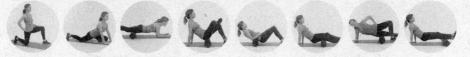

(See Chapter 15, "Flexibility and Form," for a description of the post-run stretches.)

Open High Kneel
30 seconds each leg

Low Back Stretch with Roller
45–60 seconds

Pigeon Pose
30 seconds each leg

Hamstrings Stretch with Roller
30–45 seconds each leg

Quadriceps Stretch with Roller
45–60 seconds

ITB Stretch with Roller
30–45 seconds each side

Piriformis Stretch with Roller
30–45 seconds each side

Gastrocnemius with Roller
30–35 seconds each leg

Friday: Strength-Train 15 Minutes, Stretch 10 Minutes

Strength (Resistance) Exercises (15 Minutes)

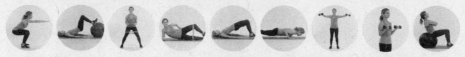

(See Chapter 14, "Strength Training for Runners," for a description of the strength exercises.)

Body-Weight Squat
30–45 seconds

Hip-Extension Leg Curl w/ Ball
20 leg curls

Lateral Step w/ Mini-Band
15 steps each side

Clamshell with Mini-Band
15–20 reps each leg

Bridge/Pelvic Thrust with Feet Flat
20 reps with pause

Push-ups (Standard or Modified)
30–45 seconds

Dumbbell Clocker Shoulder Raise
5 reps at each of the clock positions

Dumbbell Curl to Press
20 reps

Abdominal Crunch on Exercise Ball
repetitions for 60 seconds

Stretches (10 minutes)

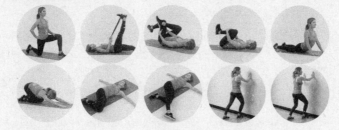

(See Chapter 15, "Flexibility and Form," for a description of the post-workout stretches.)

Tall Kneeling Stretch
30 seconds each side

Hamstrings Stretch with Rope
30 seconds each leg

Piriformis Stretch
30 seconds each side

Low Back Stretch #1
30–45 seconds

Cobra/Prone Back Extension
45 seconds

Low Back Stretch #2
30–45 seconds

Spinal Rotation Stretch
30–45 seconds each side

Hip Abductor/ITB Stretch with Spinal Rotation
30–45 seconds each side

Isolated Gastrocnemius Stretch
30 seconds each leg

Isolated Soleus Stretch
30 seconds each leg

Saturday: Dynamic Stretches 5 Minutes, Run 60–90 Minutes, Stretch 15 Minutes

Dynamic Stretches (Before Run, 5 Minutes)

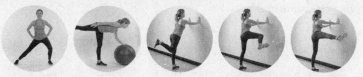

(See Chapter 15, "Flexibility and Form," for a description of the dynamic stretches.)

Dynamic Side Lunge
30 seconds each leg

Dynamic Bent-Knee Lateral Swing
10–15 reps each leg

Dynamic Single-Leg Dead Lift
30 seconds each leg

Dynamic Straight-Leg Lateral Swing
10–15 reps each leg

Dynamic Bent-Knee Forward Swing
10–15 reps each leg

Complete Key Run #3

(See Chapter 6, "Three Quality Runs," for run workouts and target times/paces.)

Stretches (After Run, 10 Minutes)

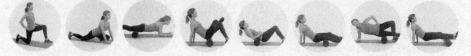

(See Chapter 15, "Flexibility and Form," for a description of the post-run stretches.)

Open High Kneel
30 seconds each leg

Low Back with Roller
45–60 seconds

Pigeon Pose
30 seconds each leg

Hamstrings Stretch with Roller
30–45 seconds each leg

Quadriceps Stretch with Roller
45–60 seconds

ITB Stretch with Roller
30–45 seconds each side

Piriformis Stretch with Roller
45 seconds each side

Gastrocnemius Stretch with Roller
30–35 seconds each leg

Sunday: Cross-Train 30 Minutes (Optional), Stretch 10 Minutes

Choose and complete any cross-training workout from Chapter 7, "Essential Cross-Training."

Stretches (10 minutes)

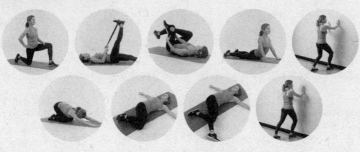

(See Chapter 15, "Flexibility and Form," for a description of the post-workout stretches.)

Tall Kneeling Stretch
30 seconds each side

Low Back Stretch #2
30–45 seconds

Hamstrings Stretch with Rope
30 seconds each leg

Spinal Rotation Stretch
30–45 seconds each side

Piriformis Stretch
30 seconds each side

Hip Abductor/ITB Stretch with Spinal Rotation
30–45 seconds each side

Cobra/Prone Back Extension
45 seconds each side

Isolated Gastrocnemius Stretch
30 seconds each leg

Isolated Soleus Stretch
30 seconds each leg

||||||

REAL RUNNER REPORT

Hi Bill and Scott,

I would like to thank you both for helping me achieve my dream of qualifying for the 2020 Boston Marathon.

After underperforming at the 2017 NYC Marathon (3:39:20), I decided that I needed to change my training plan in order to improve my performance. At this time I was running 35 miles per week across three steady paced runs, but reached a point where I was not improving.

A friend recommended getting a copy of *Run Less Run Faster*, as this would provide me with the structure for a training plan, including intervals, tempo & long run, complemented with cross-training. This gave my training more focus and complemented the limited time I had available to train.

I set myself the ambitious target of qualifying for Boston by the end of 2018, which seemed to be a long way off at the time. This structured training, coupled with some changes to my diet, has allowed me to make great improvements in my performance, which I did not think would be possible in this space of time.

Since the start of 2018, it has allowed me to improve my 5K (19:40 → 16:46), 10K (41:15 → 34:33), and HM (90:25 → 76:35) times considerably, the last of which had remained the same for six years (age 30–36). This culminated in me running a PB of 2:48:29 (previously 3:13:18) at Valencia Marathon in December 2018 and achieving my goal of qualifying for Boston.

I genuinely believe that your book was the most fundamental contributing factor to this (combined with my hard work!), so thanks again.

Best wishes,
Mark McKeown
Accountant
London, United Kingdom

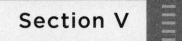
Section V

HOPKINTON OR BUST

17

The Road to Boston Is Steeper

In the 2012 edition of *Run Less Run Faster*, we reported that the road to Boston had become a little steeper, with the more stringent qualifying standards set for 2013. Because of the heavy demand from qualified runners for an entry into the Boston Marathon, the Boston Athletic Association lowered the qualifying standards in 2018 by five minutes for each age group, beginning with the 2020 Boston Marathon (Note: the marathon was cancelled due to the coronavirus pandemic). Qualifying for the Boston Marathon requires you to meet the qualifying time for your age and gender. You must do so in a certified marathon. Limits on the field size mean that meeting the qualifying standard does not guarantee entry into the race.

The fastest qualified runners are accepted until the field size limit of 30,000 runners is reached. After 2012, those accepted into the race had to better the qualifying standard by a range of 1:02 in 2015, and 4:52 in 2018. The ballooning number of qualifiers leads to disappointment for runners who meet the standard for their age group but are denied entry because accepted qualifiers have times that are faster than the standard. In 2018, that is what happened to 7,248 qualifiers for Boston.

Because of the large number of qualifiers who were not accepted into the 2019 race, the Boston Athletic Association announced in September 2018 that the qualifying standards were being updated once again. As mentioned above, the new standards lowered the qualifying time for each age group by five minutes for both men and women. Even with these stiffer qualifying standards, 3,161 runners who met the new standard were denied entry into the 2020 marathon. Qualifiers needed to have run 1:39 faster than the new standard to be accepted.

Qualifying times were instituted in 1970 to control the number of runners in the historic race that began in 1897. Boston Athletic Association officials were concerned when the race grew from 197 runners in 1960 to 1342 by 1969. It was thought that the course would become congested with more than 1000 runners. Initially, in 1970, runners had to have completed a marathon in less than four hours. That quickly changed in 1971 to 3:30. The qualifying standards have changed a dozen times since then, with the most rigorous qualifying times of 2:50 for men and 3:20 for women instituted in 1980.

Running through a corridor of cheering fans for 26.2 miles is an exhilarating experience.

I can easily understand why we receive many messages from runners who ask if we can help them qualify for Boston, the oldest and most prestigious American marathon. Because of runners' intense desires to meet the Boston qualifying standard, we have included updated Boston training plans to assist runners seeking to earn their Boston bib under the new standards. Many runners have used these plans to qualify.

Preceding each plan are our criteria for helping you determine if you have a realistic chance of meeting the standard in each plan. Attempting to qualify for Boston when the qualifying time is unrealistic for you can cause much disappointment and, perhaps, an injury. As we warn runners in Chapter 3, it's important to set realistic goals.

Ironically, trying to qualify for Boston probably causes more poor marathon performances than any other goal set by runners. Runners fall into the trap of training for too ambitious a finish time, or running too fast at the beginning of the race. Invariably, you'll suffer through the last half of the race, slowing considerably, and finish in a time slower than what your training predicted. Because of the strong desire to fulfill the popular "bucket list" of running Boston, runners are willing to risk falling apart in a qualifying marathon with hopes of defying prediction tables.

However, we believe that there is nothing more thrilling in the sport of running than the Boston Marathon. For that reason, we understand why runners are willing to risk a poor marathon experience and even injury to qualify. With that in mind, below you'll find a program that will let you know if Boston is realistic for you, and a detailed training program that will lead to a Boston bib on Patriots' Day.

How do marathoners know if their Boston qualifying times are realistic goals? Meeting the time standard, like meeting your personal goal time in any marathon, requires being properly trained for the 26.2-mile distance and having a lot of factors—personal and external—favorable on race day. Fortunately, there are some criteria that marathoners can use to determine whether they are ready for a qualifying attempt.

Judge whether your goal is realistic by using our criteria for every Boston qualifying time. Take your finish times from 5Ks, 10Ks, or half-marathon races, and see if you meet the criteria for your qualifying time. FIRST provides another method for determining if your goal is realistic: Can you run all three specified workouts for your target time for Boston in the same week?

At the end of this chapter, there are 16 sets of criteria and 16 training programs, one to match each Boston qualifying time. Young and old, male and female, there's a program for you. Meet the criteria, follow the program, and book your Boston hotel room early.

Thoughts on Marathon Training

I have said repeatedly over the past 30 years that running a marathon is a peculiar goal. What is the appeal of a 26.2-mile-distant finish line? Marathons provide us with an opportunity to challenge ourselves with a difficult goal that requires dedication of time and effort spanning months. We must remember to enjoy the journey. The marathon itself lasts only a few hours, but the anticipation is spread over several months. The weekend-long runs give runners concrete evidence of how they are getting stronger week after week as the distance of the long run increases. Having a goal that can be visualized during those 16 weeks provides an incentive for focused training and both anticipation and trepidation as the race draws near.

Marathoners often share marathon training with a friend or friends. Training partners develop deep friendships—one of the benefits of running. Experiencing a challenge with a friend makes it even more special. The social aspect of marathoning clearly has contributed to the tremendous growth in marathon participation.

I have been doubly blessed with good training partners. Coauthor Scott Murr, my brother Don, and I have shared more than 5000 training runs together. Many of the ideas for this book and its earlier edition were developed by the three of us on training runs.

Marathoners seek special destinations. Only in a marathon can you tour the monuments of Washington, DC, by running down the middle of Constitution Avenue, tour the five boroughs of New York City and experience the cheers on First Avenue, or circle the city of Chicago, running up the middle of LaSalle Street. These truly are special experiences that attract thousands of runners.

Marathoners may not always appreciate what they have accomplished when they see the finish clock at the end of their marathon effort. Unfortunately, some runners let racing become just one more source of stress in their lives. Our focus needs to be on the process and not the outcome. Training and the vitality it produces are what we need to appreciate and enjoy. Of course, we like to have racing goals, but we must remember that our race times do not define us. Training seriously and accepting the results without becoming despondent provide a positive, healthy experience. Sometimes everything seems perfect and a poor performance is inexplicable. It's this uncertainty that keeps many runners returning to the marathon, seeking that optimal performance. Because there aren't that many opportunities to run a great marathon—ideal weather combined with excellent training—marathoners keep returning to the roads for that race where all elements come together for the performance that meets their dream expectations. And when it happens, the finish line becomes drenched in emotion.

Final Comments

Running a marathon is an immensely gratifying accomplishment. Many runners have written us at FIRST, expressing their appreciation for providing them with training programs that enabled them to realize their goals of completing a marathon or qualifying for Boston. We hope you can use this book and these training programs to prepare to meet your dream challenge. Most of all, enjoy the training and make it a healthy endeavor.

For Men 18 to 34, You Must Run 3:00 to BQ

Qualifying for Boston is realistic if you can run:

a 5K in 18:30;
a 10K in 38:42; or
a half-marathon in 1:25:45 (Note: The half-marathon is the best predictor.)

If you can, complete one of each of the three Key Runs in the same week:

Key Run #1: Track repeats (complete one of the workouts listed below)
6 x 800m @ 2:43/800m with a 400m recovery jog between intervals
5 x 1000m @ 3:26/1000m with a 400m recovery jog between intervals
4 x 1200m @ 4:10/1200m with a 400m recovery jog between intervals
3 x 1600m @ 5:41/1600m with a 400m recovery jog between intervals

Key Run #2: Tempo run (complete one of the tempo runs)
After a one-mile warm-up, complete a three-mile training run in 18:42 *or*
After a 1.5km warm-up, complete a 5km training run in 19:25

After a one-mile warm-up, complete a five-mile training run in 32:25 *or*
After a 1.5km warm-up, complete an 8km training run in 32:16

After a one-mile warm-up, complete an eight-mile training run in 53:52 *or*
After a 1.5km warm-up, complete a 13km training run in 54:23

Key Run #3: Long run
Complete a 15- to 20-mile run @ 7:17/mile pace *or*
Complete a 24km to 32km run @ 4:32/km pace

3:00 Boston Marathon Training Plan

RI = Rest Interval; which may be a timed rest/recovery interval or a distance that you walk/jog.
Key Run #1 always begins with a 10–20-min warm-up and ends with a 10-min cool-down.
Key Run #2 begins and ends with a one-mile (1.5km) easy run, unless otherwise indicated.
Metric workout equivalents appear in bold italics.

WEEK	KEY RUN #1	KEY RUN #2	KEY RUN #3
16	3 x 1600 in 5:41 (400 RI)	2 miles (*3km*) easy 2 miles at 6:14 ***3km at 3:53***	13 miles at 7:22 ***21km at 4:35***
15	4 x 800 in 2:43 (2 min RI)	5 miles at 6:52 ***8km at 4:16***	15 miles at 7:37 ***24km at 4:44***
14	1200 in 4:10 (200 RI) 1000 in 3:26 (200 RI) 800 in 2:43 (200 RI) 600 in 2:01 (200 RI) 400 in 1:19 (200 RI)	5 miles at 6:44 ***8km at 4:11***	17 miles at 7:37 ***27km at 4:44***
13	5 x 1000 in 3:26 (400 RI)	4 miles at 6:29 ***7km at 4:02***	20 miles at 7:52 ***32km at 4:53***
12	3 x 1600 in 5:41 (400 RI)	2 miles (*3km*) easy 3 miles at 6:14 ***5km at 3:53***	18 miles at 7:37 ***29km at 4:44***
11	2 x 1200 in 4:10 (2 min RI) 4 x 800 in 2:43 (2 min RI)	5 miles at 6:29 ***8km at 4:02***	20 miles at 7:37 ***32km at 4:44***
10	6 x 800 in 2:43 (90 sec RI)	6 miles at 6:44 ***10km at 4:11***	13 miles at 7:07 ***21km at 4:25***
9	2 x (6 x 400 in 1:19) (90 sec RI) (2 min 30 sec RI between sets)	2 miles (*3km*) easy 3 miles at 6:14 ***5km at 3:53***	18 miles at 7:22 ***29km at 4:35***
8	2 x 1600 in 5:41 (60 sec RI) 2 x 800 in 2:43 (60 sec RI)	4 miles at 6:29 ***7km at 4:02***	20 miles at 7:22 ***32km at 4:35***
7	4 x 1200 in 4:10 (2 min RI)	10 miles at 6:52 ***16km at 4:16***	15 miles at 7:12 ***24km at 4:28***
6	1000 in 3:26, 2000 in 7:12, 1000 in 3:26, 1000 in 3:26 (400 RI)	5 miles at 6:52 ***8km at 4:16***	20 miles at 7:22 ***32km at 4:35***
5	3 x 1600 in 5:41 (400 RI)	10 miles at 6:52 ***16km at 4:16***	15 miles at 7:07 ***24km at 4:25***
4	10 x 400 in 1:19 (400 RI)	8 miles at 6:52 ***13km at 4:16***	20 miles at 7:07 ***32km at 4:25***
3	8 x 800 in 2:43 (90 sec RI)	5 miles at 6:29 ***8km at 4:02***	13 miles at 6:52 ***21km at 4:16***
2	5 x 1000 in 3:26 (400 RI)	2 miles (*3km*) easy 3 miles at 6:14 ***5km at 3:53***	10 miles at 6:52 ***16km at 4:16***
1	6 x 400 in 1:19 (400 RI)	3 miles at 6:52 ***5km at 4:16***	MARATHON 26.2 miles at 6:52 ***42.2km at 4:16***

For Men 35 to 39, You Must Run 3:05 to BQ

Qualifying for Boston is realistic if you can run:

a 5K in 19:00;
a 10K in 39:45; or
a half-marathon in 1:28:04. (Note: The half-marathon is the best predictor.)

If you can, complete one of each of the three Key Runs in the same week:

Key Run #1: Track repeats (complete one of the workouts listed below)
6 x 800m @ 2:47/800m with a 400m recovery jog between intervals
5 x 1000m @ 3:32/1000m with a 400m recovery jog between intervals
4 x 1200m @ 4:17/1200m with a 400m recovery jog between intervals
3 x 1600m @ 5:51/1600m with a 400m recovery jog between intervals

Key Run #2: Tempo run (complete one of the tempo runs)
After a one-mile warm-up, complete a three-mile training run in 19:12 *or*
After a 1.5km warm-up, complete a 5km training run in 19:55

After a one-mile warm-up, complete a five-mile training run in 33:15 *or*
After a 1.5km warm-up, complete an 8km training run in 33:04

After a one-mile warm-up, complete an eight-mile training run in 55:12 *or*
After a 1.5km warm-up, complete a 13km training run in 55:41

Key Run #3: Long run
Complete a 15- to 20-mile run @ 7:28/mile pace *or*
Complete a 24km to 32km run @ 4:38/km pace

3:05 Boston Marathon Training Plan

RI = Rest Interval; which may be a timed rest/recovery interval or a distance that you walk/jog.
Key Run #1 always begins with a 10–20-min warm-up and ends with a 10-min cool-down.
Key Run #2 begins and ends with a one-mile (1.5km) easy run, unless otherwise indicated.
Metric workout equivalents appear in bold italics.

WEEK	KEY RUN #1	KEY RUN #2	KEY RUN #3
16	3 x 1600 in 5:51 (400 RI)	2 miles (*3km*) Easy 2 miles at 6:24 ***3km at 3:59*** 2 miles (3K) Easy	13 miles at 7:33 ***21km at 4:42***
15	4 x 800 in 2:47 (2 min RI)	5 miles at 7:03 ***8km at 4:23***	15 miles at 7:48 ***24km at 4:51***
14	1200 in 4:17 (200 RI) 1000 in 3:32 (200 RI) 800 in 2:47 (200 RI) 600 in 2:05 (200 RI) 400 in 1:22 (200 RI)	5 miles at 6:54 ***8km at 4:17***	17 miles at 7:48 ***27km at 4:51***
13	5 x 1000 in 3:32 (400 RI)	4 miles at 6:39 ***7km at 4:08***	20 miles at 8:03 ***32km at 5:00***
12	3 x 1600 in 5:51 (400 RI)	2 miles (*3km*) Easy 3 miles at 6:24 ***5km at 3:59***	18 miles at 7:48 ***29km at 4:51***
11	2 x 1200 in 4:17 (2 min RI) 4 x 800 in 2:47 (2 min RI)	5 miles at 6:39 ***8km at 4:08***	20 miles at 7:48 ***32km at 4:51***
10	6 x 800 in 2:47 (90 sec RI)	6 miles at 6:54 ***10km at 4:17***	13 miles at 7:18 ***21km at 4:32***
9	2 x (6x 400 in 1:22) (90 sec RI) (2 min 30 sec RI between sets)	2 miles (*3km*) Easy 3 miles at 6:24 ***5km at 3:59***	18 miles at 7:33 ***29km at 4:42***
8	2 x 1600 in 5:51 (60 sec RI) 2 x 800 in 2:47 (60 sec RI)	4 miles at 6:39 ***7km at 4:08***	20 miles at 7:33 ***32km at 4:42***
7	4 x 1200 in 4:17 (2 min RI)	10 miles at 7:03 ***16km at 4:23***	15 miles at 7:23 ***24km at 4:35***
6	1000 in 3:32, 2000 in 7:24, 1000 in 3:32, 1000 in 3:32 (400 RI)	5 miles at 7:03 ***8km at 4:23***	20 miles at 7:33 ***32km at 4:42***
5	3 x 1600 in 5:51 (400 RI)	10 miles at 7:03 ***16km at 4:23***	15 miles at 7:18 ***24km at 4:32***
4	10 x 400 in 1:22 (400 RI)	8 miles at 7:03 ***13km at 4:23***	20 miles at 7:18 ***32km at 4:32***
3	8 x 800 in 2:47 (90 sec RI)	5 miles at 6:39 ***8km at 4:08***	13 miles at 7:03 ***21km at 4:23***
2	5 x 1000 in 3:32 (400 RI)	2 miles (*3km*) Easy 3 miles at 6:24 ***5km at 3:59***	10 miles at 7:03 ***16km at 4:23***
1	6 x 400 in 1:22 (400 RI)	3 miles at 7:03 ***5km at 4:23***	MARATHON 26.2 miles at 7:03 ***42.2km at 4:23***

For Men 40 to 44, You Must Run 3:10 to BQ

Qualifying for Boston is realistic if you can run:

a 5K in 19:30;
a 10K in 40:48; or
a half-marathon in 1:30:23. (Note: The half-marathon is the best predictor.)

If you can, complete one of each of the three Key Runs in the same week:

Key Run #1: Track repeats (complete one of the workouts listed below)
6 x 800m @ 2:52/800m with a 400m recovery jog between intervals
5 x 1000m @ 3:38/1000m with a 400m recovery jog between intervals
4 x 1200m @ 4:24/1200m with a 400m recovery jog between intervals
3 x 1600m @ 6:01/1600m with a 400m recovery jog between intervals

Key Run #2: Tempo run (complete one of the tempo runs)
After a one-mile warm-up, complete a three-mile training run in 19:42 *or*
After a 1.5km warm-up, complete a 5km training run in 20:25

After a one-mile warm-up, complete a five-mile training run in 34:05 *or*
After a 1.5km warm-up, complete an 8km training run in 33:52

After a one-mile warm-up, complete an eight-mile training run in 56:32 *or*
After a 1.5km warm-up, complete a 13km training run in 57:00

Key Run #3: Long run
Complete a 15- to 20-mile run @ 7:39/mile pace *or*
Complete a 24km to 32km run @ 4:45/km pace

3:10 Boston Marathon Training Plan

RI = Rest Interval; which may be a timed rest/recovery interval or a distance that you walk/jog.
Key Run #1 always begins with a 10–20-min warm-up and ends with a 10-min cool-down.
Key Run #2 begins and ends with a one-mile (1.5km) easy run, unless otherwise indicated.
Metric workout equivalents appear in bold italics.

WEEK	KEY RUN #1	KEY RUN #2	KEY RUN #3
16	3 x 1600 in 6:01 (400 RI)	2 miles (*3km*) Easy 2 miles at 6:34 ***3km at 4:05*** 2 miles (*3km*) Easy	13 miles at 7:44 ***21km at 4:49***
15	4 x 800 in 2:52 (2 min RI)	5 miles at 7:14 ***8km at 4:30***	15 miles at 7:59 ***24km at 4:58***
14	1200 in 4:24 (200 RI) 1000 in 3:38 (200 RI) 800 in 2:52 (200 RI) 600 in 2:08 (200 RI) 400 in 1:24 (200 RI)	5 miles at 7:04 ***8km at 4:23***	17 miles at 7:59 ***27km at 4:58***
13	5 x 1000 in 3:38 (400 RI)	4 miles at 6:49 ***7km at 4:14***	20 miles at 8:14 ***32km at 5:07***
12	3 x 1600 in 6:01 (400 RI)	2 miles (*3km*) Easy 3 miles at 6:34 ***5km at 4:05***	18 miles at 7:59 ***29km at 4:58***
11	2 x 1200 in 4:24 (2 min RI) 4 x 800 in 2:52 (2 min RI)	5 miles at 6:49 ***8km at 4:14***	20 miles at 7:59 ***32km at 4:58***
10	6 x 800 in 2:52 (90 sec RI)	6 miles at 7:04 ***10km at 4:23***	13 miles at 7:29 ***21km at 4:39***
9	2 x (6x 400 in 1:24) (90 sec RI) (2 min 30 sec RI between sets)	2 miles (*3km*) Easy 3 miles at 6:34 ***5km at 4:05***	18 miles at 7:44 ***29km at 4:49***
8	2 x 1600 In 6:01 (60 sec RI) 2 x 800 in 2:52 (60 sec RI)	4 miles at 6:49 ***7km at 4:14***	20 miles at 7:44 ***32km at 4:49***
7	4 x 1200 in 4:24 (2 min RI)	10 miles at 7:14 ***16km at 4:30***	15 miles at 7:34 ***24km at 4:42***
6	1000 in 3:38, 2000 In 7:36, 1000 in 3:38, 1000 in 3:38 (400 RI)	5 miles at 7:14 ***8km at 4:30***	20 mlles at 7:44 ***32km at 4:49***
5	3 x 1600 in 6:01 (400 RI)	10 miles at 7:14 ***16km at 4:30***	15 miles at 7:29 ***24km at 4:39***
4	10 x 400 in 1:24 (400 RI)	8 miles at 7:14 ***13km at 4:30***	20 miles at 7:29 ***32km at 4:39***
3	8 x 800 in 2:52 (90 sec RI)	5 miles at 6:49 ***8km at 4:14***	13 miles at 7:14 ***21km at 4:30***
2	5 x 1000 in 3:38 (400 RI)	2 miles (*3km*) Easy 3 miles at 6:34 ***5km at 4:06***	10 miles at 7:14 ***16km at 4:30***
1	6 x 400 in 1:24 (400 RI)	3 miles at 7:14 ***5km at 4:30***	MARATHON 26.2 miles at 7:14 ***42.2km at 4:30***

For Men 45 to 49, You Must Run 3:20 to BQ

Qualifying for Boston is realistic if you can run:

a 5K in 20:33;
a 10K in 43:00; or
a half-marathon in 1:35:16. (Note: The half-marathon is the best predictor.)

If you can, complete one of each of the three Key Runs in the same week:

Key Run #1: Track repeats (complete one of the workouts listed below)
6 x 800m @ 3:02/800m with a 400m recovery jog between intervals
5 x 1000m @ 3:50/1000m with a 400m recovery jog between intervals
4 x 1200m @ 4:40/1200m with a 400m recovery jog between intervals
3 x 1600m @ 6:21/1600m with a 400m recovery jog between intervals

Key Run #2: Tempo run (complete one of the tempo runs)
After a one-mile warm-up, complete a three-mile training run in 20:42 *or*
After a 1.5km warm-up, complete a 5km training run in 21:25

After a one-mile warm-up, complete a five-mile training run in 35:45 *or*
After a 1.5km warm-up, complete an 8km training run in 35:36

After a one-mile warm-up, complete an eight-mile training run in 59:12 *or*
After a 1.5km warm-up, complete a 13km training run in 59:48

Key Run #3: Long run
Complete a 15- to 20-mile run @ 8:03/mile pace *or*
Complete a 24km to 32km run @ 5:00/km pace

3:20 Boston Marathon Training Plan

RI = Rest Interval; which may be a timed rest/recovery interval or a distance that you walk/jog.
Key Run #1 always begins with a 10–20 min warm-up and ends with a 10-min cool-down.
Key Run #2 begins and ends with a one-mile (1.5K) easy run, unless otherwise indicated.
Metric workout equivalents appear in bold italics.

WEEK	KEY RUN #1	KEY RUN #2	KEY RUN #3
16	3 x 1600 in 6:21 (400 RI)	2 miles (*3km*) Easy 2 miles at 6:54 *3km at 4:17* 2 miles (*3km*) Easy	13 miles at 8:07 *21km at 5:03*
15	4 x 800 in 3:02 (2 min RI)	5 miles at 7:37 *8km at 4:44*	15 miles at 8:22 *24km at 5:12*
14	1200 in 4:40 (200 RI) 1000 in 3:50 (200 RI) 800 in 3:02 (200 RI) 600 in 2:16 (200 RI) 400 in 1:29 (200 RI)	5 miles at 7:24 *8km at 4:36*	17 miles at 8:22 *27km at 5:12*
13	5 x 1000 in 3:50 (400 RI)	4 miles at 7:09 *7km at 4:27*	20 miles at 8:37 *32km at 5:21*
12	3 x 1600 in 6:21 (400 RI)	2 miles (*3km*) Easy 3 miles at 6:54 *5km at 4:17*	18 miles at 8:22 *29km at 5:12*
11	2 x 1200 in 4:40 (2 min RI) 4 x 800 in 3:02 (2 min RI)	5 miles at 7:09 *8km at 4:27*	20 miles at 8:22 *32km at 5:12*
10	6 x 800 in 3:02 (90 sec RI)	6 miles at 7:24 *10km at 4:36*	13 miles at 7:52 *21km at 4:53*
9	2 x (6x 400 in 1:29) (90 sec RI) (2 min 30 sec RI between sets)	2 miles (*3km*) Easy 3 miles at 6:54 *5km at 4:17*	18 miles at 8:07 *29km at 5:03*
8	2 x 1600 in 6:21 (60 sec RI) 2 x 800 in 3:02 (60 sec RI)	4 miles at 7:09 *7km at 4:27*	20 miles at 8:07 *32km at 5:03*
7	4 x 1200 in 4:40 (2 min RI)	10 miles at 7:37 *16km at 4:44*	15 miles at 7:57 *24km at 4:56*
6	1000 in 3:50, 2000 in 8:01, 1000 in 3:50, 1000 in 3:50 (400 RI)	5 miles at 7:37 *8km at 4:44*	20 miles at 8:07 *32km at 5:03*
5	3 x 1600 in 6:21 (400 RI)	10 miles at 7:37 *16km at 4:44*	15 miles at 7:52 *24km at 4:53*
4	10 x 400 in 1:29 (400 RI)	8 miles at 7:37 *13km at 4:44*	20 miles at 7:52 *32km at 4:53*
3	8 x 800 in 3:02 (90 sec RI)	5 miles at 7:09 *8km at 4:27*	13 miles at 7:37 *21km at 4:44*
2	5 x 1000 in 3:50 (400 RI)	2 miles (*3km*) Easy 3 miles at 6:54 *5km at 4:17*	10 miles at 7:37 *16km at 4:44*
1	6 x 400 in 1:29 (400 RI)	3 miles at 7:37 *5km at 4:44*	MARATHON 26.2 miles at 7:37 *42.2km at 4:44*

For Men 50 to 54, You Must Run 3:25 to BQ

Qualifying for Boston is realistic if you can run:

a 5K in 21:05;
a 10K in 44:06; or
a half-marathon in 1:37:25. (Note: The half-marathon is the best predictor.)

If you can, complete one of each of the three Key Runs in the same week:

Key Run #1: Track repeats (complete one of the workouts listed below)
6 x 800m @ 3:08/800m with a 400m recovery jog between intervals
5 x 1000m @ 3:56/1000m with a 400m recovery jog between intervals
4 x 1200m @ 4:47/1200m with a 400m recovery jog between intervals
3 x 1600m @ 6:31/1600m with a 400m recovery jog between intervals

Key Run #2: Tempo run (complete one of the tempo runs)
After a one-mile warm-up, complete a three-mile training run in 21:12 *or*
After a 1.5km warm-up, complete a 5km training run in 22:00

After a one-mile warm-up, complete a five-mile training run in 36:35 *or*
After a 1.5km warm-up, complete an 8km training run in 36:24

After a one-mile warm-up, complete an eight-mile training run in 60:32 *or*
After a 1.5km warm-up, complete a 13km training run in 61:06

Key Run #3: Long run
Complete a 15- to 20-mile run @ 8:15/mile pace *or*
Complete a 24km to 32km run @ 5:07/km pace

3:25 Boston Marathon Training Plan

RI = Rest Interval; which may be a timed rest/recovery interval or a distance that you walk/jog.
Key Run #1 always begins with a 10–20-min warm-up and ends with a 10-min cool-down.
Key Run #2 begins and ends with a one-mile (1.5km) easy run, unless otherwise indicated.
Metric workout equivalents appear in bold italics.

WEEK	KEY RUN #1	KEY RUN #2	KEY RUN #3
16	3 x 1600 in 6:31 (400 RI)	2 miles (*3km*) Easy 2 miles at 7:04 ***3km at 4:24*** 2 miles (*3km*) Easy	13 miles at 8:19 ***21km at 5:10***
15	4 x 800 in 3:08 (2 min RI)	5 miles at 7:49 ***8km at 4:51***	15 miles at 8:34 ***24km at 5:19***
14	1200 in 4:47 (200 RI) 1000 in 3:56 (200 RI) 800 in 3:08 (200 RI) 600 in 2:20 (200 RI) 400 in 1:32 (200 RI)	5 miles at 7:34 ***8km at 4:42***	17 miles at 8:34 ***27km at 5:19***
13	5 x 1000 in 3:56 (400 RI)	4 miles at 7:19 ***7km at 4:33***	20 miles at 8:49 ***32km at 5:28***
12	3 x 1600 in 6:31 (400 RI)	2 miles (*3km*) Easy 3 miles at 7:04 ***5km at 4:24***	18 miles at 8:34 ***29km at 5:19***
11	2 x 1200 in 4:47 (2 min RI) 4 x 800 in 3:08 (2 min RI)	5 miles at 7:19 ***8km at 4:33***	20 miles at 8:34 ***32km at 5:19***
10	6 x 800 in 3:08 (90 sec RI)	6 miles at 7:34 ***10km at 4:42***	13 miles at 8:04 ***21km at 5:00***
9	2 x (6x 400 in 1:32) (90 sec RI) (2 min 30 sec RI between sets)	2 miles (*3km*) Easy 3 miles at 7:04 ***5km at 4:24***	18 miles at 8:19 ***29km at 5:10***
8	2 x 1600 in 6:31 (60 sec RI) 2 x 800 in 3:08 (60 sec RI)	4 miles at 7:19 ***7km at 4:33***	20 miles at 8:19 ***32km at 5:10***
7	3 x (2 x 1200 in 4:47) (2 min RI) (4 min RI between sets)	10 miles at 7:49 ***16km at 4:51***	15 miles at 8:09 ***24km at 5:03***
6	1000 in 3:56, 2000 in 8:14, 1000 in 3:56, 1000 in 3:56 (400 RI)	5 miles at 7:49 ***8km at 4:51***	20 miles at 8:19 ***32km at 5:10***
5	3 x 1600 in 6:31 (400 RI)	10 miles at 7:49 ***16km at 4:51***	15 miles at 8:04 ***24km at 5:00***
4	10 x 400 in 1:32 (400 RI)	8 miles at 7:49 ***13km at 4:51***	20 miles at 8:04 ***32km at 5:00***
3	8 x 800 in 3:08 (90 sec RI)	5 miles at 7:19 ***8km at 4:33***	13 miles at 7:49 ***21km at 4:51***
2	5 x 1000 in 3:56 (400 RI)	2 miles (*3km*) Easy 3 miles at 7:04 ***5km at 4:24***	10 miles at 7:49 ***16km at 4:51***
1	6 x 400 in 1:32 (400 RI)	3 miles at 7:49 ***5km at 4:51***	MARATHON 26.2 miles at 7:49 ***42.2km at 4:51***

For Women 18 to 34, You Must Run 3:30 to BQ

Qualifying for Boston is realistic if you can run:

a 5K in 21:35;
a 10K in 45:10; or
a half-marathon in 1:40:00. (Note: The half-marathon is the best predictor.)

If you can, complete one of each of the three Key Runs in the same week:

Key Run #1: Track repeats (complete one of the workouts listed below)
6 x 800m @ 3:12/800m with a 400m recovery jog between intervals
5 x 1000m @ 4:02/1000m with a 400m recovery jog between intervals
4 x 1200m @ 4:55/1200m with a 400m recovery jog between intervals
3 x 1600m @ 6:41/1600m with a 400m recovery jog between intervals

Key Run #2: Tempo run (complete one of the tempo runs)
After a one-mile warm-up, complete a three-mile training run in 21:42 *or*
After a 1.5km warm-up, complete a 5km training run in 22:30

After a one-mile warm-up, complete a five-mile training run in 37:25 *or*
After a 1.5km warm-up, complete an 8km training run in 37:12

After a one-mile warm-up, complete an eight-mile training run in 61:52 *or*
After a 1.5km warm-up, complete a 13km training run in 62:24

Key Run #3: Long run
Complete a 15- to 20-mile run @ 8:25/mile pace *or*
Complete a 24km to 32km run @ 5:15/km pace

3:30 Boston Marathon Training Plan

RI = Rest Interval; which may be a timed rest/recovery interval or a distance that you walk/jog.
Key Run #1 always begins with a 10–20-min warm-up and ends with a 10-min cool-down.
Key Run #2 begins and ends with a one-mile (1.5km) easy run, unless otherwise indicated.
Metric workout equivalents appear in bold italics.

WEEK	KEY RUN #1	KEY RUN #2	KEY RUN #3
16	3 x 1600 in 6:41 (400 RI)	2 miles (*3km*) Easy 2 miles at 7:14 ***3km at 4:30*** 2 miles (*3km*) Easy	13 miles at 8:30 ***21km at 5:17***
15	4 x 800 in 3:12 (2 min RI)	5 miles at 8:00 ***8km at 4:59***	15 miles at 8:45 ***24km at 5:26***
14	1200 in 4:55 (200 RI) 1000 in 4:02 (200 RI) 800 in 3:12 (200 RI) 600 in 2:23 (200 RI) 400 in 1:34 (200 RI)	5 miles at 7:44 ***8km at 4:48***	17 miles at 8:45 ***27km at 5:26***
13	5 x 1000 in 4:02 (400 RI)	4 miles at 7:29 ***7km at 4:39***	20 miles at 9:00 ***32km at 5:35***
12	3 x 1600 in 6:41 (400 RI)	2 miles (*3km*) Easy 3 miles at 7:14 ***5km at 4:30***	18 miles at 8:45 ***29km at 5:26***
11	2 x 1200 in 4:55 (2 min RI) 4 x 800 in 3:12 (2 min RI)	5 miles at 7:29 ***8km at 4:39***	20 miles at 8:45 ***32km at 5:26***
10	6 x 800 in 3:12 (90 sec RI)	6 miles at 7:44 ***10km at 4:48***	13 miles at 8:15 ***21km at 5:07***
9	2 x (6x 400 in 1:34) (90 sec RI) (2 min 30 sec RI between sets)	2 miles (*3km*) Easy 3 miles at 7:14 ***5km at 4:30***	18 miles at 8:30 ***29km at 5:17***
8	2 x 1600 in 6:41 (60 sec RI) 2 x 800 in 3:12 (60 sec RI)	4 miles at 7:29 ***7km at 4:39***	20 miles at 8:30 ***32km at 5:17***
7	4 x 1200 in 4:55 (2 min RI) (4 min RI between sets)	10 miles at 8:00 ***16km at 4:58***	15 miles at 8:20 ***24km at 5:10***
6	1000 in 4:02, 2000 in 8:26, 1000 in 4:02, 1000 in 4:02 (400 RI)	5 miles at 8:00 ***8km at 4:58***	20 miles at 8:30 ***32km at 5:17***
5	3 x 1600 in 6:41 (400 RI)	10 miles at 8:00 ***16km at 4:58***	15 miles at 8:15 ***24km at 5:07***
4	10 x 400 in 1:34 (400 RI)	8 miles at 8:00 ***13km at 4:58***	20 miles at 8:15 ***32km at 5:07***
3	8 x 800 in 3:12 (90 sec RI)	5 miles at 7:29 ***8km at 4:39***	13 miles at 8:00 ***21km at 4:58***
2	5 x 1000 in 4:02 (400 RI)	2 miles (*3km*) Easy 3 miles at 7:14 ***5km at 4:30***	10 miles at 8:00 ***16km at 4:58***
1	6 x 400 in 1:34 (400 RI)	3 miles at 8:00 ***5km at 4:58***	MARATHON 26.2 miles at 8:00 ***42.2km at 4:58***

For Men 55 to 59 and Women 35 to 39, You Must Run 3:35 to BQ

Qualifying for Boston is realistic if you can run:

a 5K in 22:05;
a 10K in 46:10; or
a half-marathon in 1:42:20. (Note: The half-marathon is the best predictor.)

If you can, complete one of each of the three Key Runs in the same week:

Key Run #1: Track repeats (complete one of the workouts listed below)
6 x 800m @ 3:17/800m with a 400m recovery jog between intervals
5 x 1000m @ 4:09/1000m with a 400m recovery jog between intervals
4 x 1200m @ 5:02/1200m with a 400m recovery jog between intervals
3 x 1600m @ 6:50/1600m with a 400m recovery jog between intervals

Key Run #2: Tempo run (complete one of the tempo runs)
After a one-mile warm-up, complete a three-mile training run in 22:09 *or*
After a 1.5km warm-up, complete a 5km training run in 23:00

After a one-mile warm-up, complete a five-mile training run in 38:10 *or*
After a 1.5km warm-up, complete an 8km training run in 38:00

After a one-mile warm-up, complete an eight-mile training run in 63:04 *or*
After a 1.5km warm-up, complete a 13km training run in 63:42

Key Run #3: Long run
Complete a 15- to 20-mile run @ 8:37/mile pace *or*
Complete a 24km to 32km run @ 5:20/km pace

3:35 Boston Marathon Training Plan

RI = Rest Interval; which may be a timed rest/recovery interval or a distance that you walk/jog.
Key Run #1 always begins with a 10–20-min warm-up and ends with a 10-min cool-down.
Key Run #2 begins and ends with a one-mile (1.5km) easy run, unless otherwise indicated.
Metric workout equivalents appear in bold italics.

WEEK	KEY RUN #1	KEY RUN #2	KEY RUN #3
16	3 x 1600 in 6:51 (400 RI)	2 miles (*3km*) Easy 2 miles at 7:23 *3km at 4:35* 2 miles (*3km*) Easy	13 miles at 8:42 *21km at 5:24*
15	4 x 800 in 3:17 (2 min RI)	5 miles at 8:12 *8km at 5:05*	15 miles at 8:57 *24km at 5:33*
14	1200 in 5:02 (200 RI) 1000 in 4:09 (200 RI) 800 in 3:17 (200 RI) 600 in 2:27 (200 RI) 400 in 1:37 (200 RI)	5 miles at 7:53 *8km at 4:54*	17 miles at 8:57 *27km at 5:33*
13	5 x 1000 in 4:09 (400 RI)	4 miles at 7:38 *7km at 4:45*	20 miles at 9:12 *32km at 5:42*
12	3 x 1600 in 6:51 (400 RI)	2 miles (*3km*) Easy 3 miles at 7:23 *5km at 4:35*	18 miles at 8:57 *29km at 5:33*
11	2 x 1200 in 5:02 (2 min RI) 4 x 800 in 3:17 (2 min RI)	5 miles at 7:38 *8km at 4:45*	20 miles at 8:57 *32km at 5:33*
10	6 x 800 in 3:17 (90 sec RI)	6 miles at 7:53 *10km at 4:54*	13 miles at 8:27 *21km at 5:14*
9	2 x (6x 400 in 1:37) (90 sec RI) (2 min 30 sec RI between sets)	2 miles (*3km*) Easy 3 miles at 7:23 *5km at 4:35*	18 miles at 8:42 *29km at 5:24*
8	2 x 1600 in 6:51 (60 sec RI) 2 x 800 in 3:17 (60 sec RI)	4 miles at 7:38 *7km at 4:45*	20 miles at 8:42 *32km at 5:24*
7	4 x 1200 in 5:02 (2 min RI) (4 min RI between sets)	10 miles at 8:12 *16km at 5:05*	15 miles at 8:32 *24km at 5:17*
6	1000 in 4:09, 2000 in 8:38, 1000 in 4:09, 1000 in 4:09 (400 RI)	5 miles at 8:12 *8km at 5:05*	20 miles at 8:42 *32km at 5:24*
5	3 x 1600 in 6:51 (400 RI)	10 miles at 8:12 *16km at 5:05*	15 miles at 8:27 *24km at 5:14*
4	10 x 400 in 1:37 (400 RI)	8 miles at 8:12 *13km at 5:05*	20 miles at 8:27 *32km at 5:14*
3	8 x 800 in 3:17 (90 sec RI)	5 miles at 7:38 *8km at 4:45*	13 miles at 8:12 *21km at 5:05*
2	5 x 1000 in 4:09 (400 RI)	2 miles (*3km*) Easy 3 miles at 7:23 *5km at 4:35*	10 miles at 8:12 *16km at 5:05*
1	6 x 400 in 1:37 (400 RI)	3 miles at 8:12 *5km at 5:05*	MARATHON 26.2 miles at 8:12 *42.2km at 5:05*

For Women 40 to 44, You Must Run 3:40 to BQ

Qualifying for Boston is realistic if you can run:

a 5K in 22:37;
a 10K in 47:18; or
a half-marathon in 1:44:49. (Note: The half-marathon is the best predictor.)

If you can, complete one of each of the three Key Runs in the same week:

Key Run #1: Track repeats (complete one of the workouts listed below)
6 x 800m @ 3:22/800m with a 400m recovery jog between intervals
5 x 1000m @ 4:16/1000m with a 400m recovery jog between intervals
4 x 1200m @ 5:10/1200m with a 400m recovery jog between intervals
3 x 1600m @ 7:01/1600m with a 400m recovery jog between intervals

Key Run #2: Tempo run (complete one of the tempo runs)
After a one-mile warm-up, complete a three-mile training run in 22:42 *or*
After a 1.5km warm-up, complete a 5km training run in 23:30

After a one-mile warm-up, complete a five-mile training run in 39:05 *or*
After a 1.5km warm-up, complete an 8km training run in 38:48

After a one-mile warm-up, complete an eight-mile training run in 64:32 *or*
After a 1.5km warm-up, complete a 13km training run in 65:13

Key Run #3: Long run
Complete a 15- to 20-mile run @ 8:49/mile pace *or*
Complete a 24km to 32km run @ 5:29/km pace

3:40 Boston Marathon Training Plan

RI = Rest Interval; which may be a timed rest/recovery interval or a distance that you walk/jog.
Key Run #1 always begins with a 10–20-min warm-up and ends with a 10-min cool-down.
Key Run #2 begins and ends with a one-mile (1.5km) easy run, unless otherwise indicated.
Metric workout equivalents appear in bold italics.

WEEK	KEY RUN #1	KEY RUN #2	KEY RUN #3
16	3 x 1600 in 7:01 (400 RI)	2 miles (*3km*) Easy 2 miles at 7:34 ***3km at 4:41*** 2 miles (*3km*) Easy	13 miles at 8:53 ***21km at 5:31***
15	4 x 800 in 3:22 (2 min RI)	5 miles at 8:23 ***8km at 5:12***	15 miles at 9:08 ***24km at 5:40***
14	1200 in 5:10 (200 RI) 1000 in 4:16 (200 RI) 800 in 3:22 (200 RI) 600 in 2:31 (200 RI) 400 in 1:39 (200 RI)	5 miles at 8:04 ***8km at 5:01***	17 miles at 9:08 ***27km at 5:40***
13	5 x 1000 in 4:16 (400 RI)	4 miles at 7:49 ***7km at 4:51***	20 miles at 9:23 ***32km at 5:49***
12	3 x 1600 in 7:01 (400 RI)	2 miles (*3km*) Easy 3 miles at 7:34 ***5km at 4:41***	18 miles at 9:08 ***29km at 5:40***
11	2 x 1200 in 5:10 (2 min RI) 4 x 800 in 3:22 (2 min RI)	5 miles at 7:49 ***8km at 4:51***	20 miles at 9:08 ***32km at 5:40***
10	6 x 800 in 3:22 (90 sec RI)	6 miles at 8:04 ***10km at 5:01***	13 miles at 8:38 ***21km at 5:21***
9	2 x (6x 400 in 1:39) (90 sec RI) (2 min 30 sec RI between sets)	2 miles (*3km*) Easy 3 miles at 7:34 ***5km at 4:41***	18 miles at 8:53 ***29km at 5:31***
8	2 x 1600 in 7:01 (60 sec RI) 2 x 800 in 3:22 (60 sec RI)	4 miles at 7:49 ***7km at 4:51***	20 miles at 8:53 ***32km at 5:31***
7	4 x 1200 in 5:10 (2 min RI) (4 min RI between sets)	10 miles at 8:23 ***16km at 5:12***	15 miles at 8:43 ***24km at 5:24***
6	1000 in 4:16, 2000 in 8:51, 1000 in 4:16, 1000 in 4:16 (400 RI)	5 miles at 8:23 ***8km at 5:12***	20 miles at 8:53 ***32km at 5:31***
5	3 x 1600 in 7:01 (400 RI)	10 miles at 8:23 ***16km at 5:12***	15 miles at 8:38 ***24km at 5:21***
4	10 x 400 in 1:39 (400 RI)	8 miles at 8:23 ***13km at 5:12***	20 miles at 8:38 ***32km at 5:21***
3	8 x 800 in 3:22 (90 sec RI)	5 miles at 7:49 ***8km at 4:51***	13 miles at 8:23 ***21km at 5:12***
2	5 x 1000 in 4:16 (400 RI)	2 miles (*3km*) Easy 3 miles at 7:34 ***5km at 4:41***	10 miles at 8:23 ***16km at 5:12***
1	6 x 400 in 1:39 (400 RI)	3 miles at 8:23 ***5km at 5:12***	MARATHON 26.2 miles at 8:23 ***42.2km at 5:12***

For Men 60 to 64 and Women 45 to 49, You Must Run 3:50 to BQ

Qualifying for Boston is realistic if you can run:

a 5K in 23:40;
a 10K in 49:31; or
a half-marathon in 1:49:42. (Note: The half-marathon is the best predictor.)

If you can, complete one of each of the three Key Runs in the same week:

Key Run #1: Track repeats (complete one of the workouts listed below)
6 x 800m @ 3:33/800m with a 400m recovery jog between intervals
5 x 1000m @ 4:27/1000m with a 400m recovery jog between intervals
4 x 1200m @ 5:26/1200m with a 400m recovery jog between intervals
3 x 1600m @ 7:21/1600m with a 400m recovery jog between intervals

Key Run #2: Tempo run (complete one of the tempo runs)
After a one-mile warm-up, complete a three-mile training run in 23:42 *or*
After a 1.5km warm-up, complete a 5km training run in 24:35

After a one-mile warm-up, complete a five-mile training run in 40:45 *or*
After a 1.5km warm-up, complete an 8km training run in 40:32

After a one-mile warm-up, complete an eight-mile training run in 67:12 *or*
After a 1.5km warm-up, complete a 13km training run in 67:49

Key Run #3: Long run
Complete a 15- to 20-mile run @ 9:12/mile pace *or*
Complete a 24km to 32km run @ 5:43/km pace

3:50 Boston Marathon Training Plan

RI = Rest Interval; which may be a timed rest/recovery interval or a distance that you walk/jog.
Key Run #1 always begins with a 10–20-min warm-up and ends with a 10-min cool-down.
Key Run #2 begins and ends with a one-mile (1.5km) easy run, unless otherwise indicated.
Metric workout equivalents appear in bold italics.

WEEK	KEY RUN #1	KEY RUN #2	KEY RUN #3
16	3 x 1600 in 7:19 (400 RI)	2 miles (*3km*) Easy 2 miles at 7:52 ***3km at 4:53*** 2 miles (3K) Easy	13 miles at 9:16 ***21km at 5:46***
15	4 x 800 in 3:32 (2 min RI)	5 miles at 8:46 ***8km at 5:27***	15 miles at 9:31 ***24km at 5:55***
14	1200 in 5:26 (200 RI) 1000 in 4:27 (200 RI) 800 in 3:32 (200 RI) 600 in 2:38 (200 RI) 400 in 1:44 (200 RI)	5 miles at 8:24 ***8km at 5:13***	17 miles at 9:31 ***27km at 5:55***
13	5 x 1000 in 4:27 (400 RI)	4 miles at 8:07 ***7km at 5:03***	20 miles at 9:46 ***32km at 6:04***
12	3 x 1600 in 7:19 (400 RI)	2 miles (*3km*) Easy 3 miles at 7:52 ***5km at 4:53***	18 miles at 9:31 ***29km at 5:55***
11	2 x 1200 in 5:26 (2 min RI) 4 x 800 in 3:32 (2 min RI)	5 miles at 8:07 ***8km at 5:03***	20 miles at 9:31 ***32km at 5:55***
10	6 x 800 in 3:32 (90 sec RI)	6 miles at 8:24 ***10km at 5:13***	13 miles at 9:01 ***21km at 5:36***
9	2 x (6x 400 in 1:44) (90 sec RI) (2 min 30 sec RI between sets)	2 miles (*3km*) Easy 3 miles at 7:52 ***5km at 4:53***	18 miles at 9:16 ***29km at 5:46***
8	2 x 1600 in 7:19(60 sec RI) 2 x 800 in 3:32 (60 sec RI)	4 miles at 8:07 ***7km at 5:03***	20 miles at 9:16 ***32km at 5:46***
7	4 x 1200 in 5:26 (2 min RI) (4 min RI between sets)	10 miles at 8:46 ***16km at 5:27***	15 miles at 9:06 ***24km at 5:39***
6	1000 in 4:27, 2000 in 9:16, 1000 in 4:27, 1000 in 4:27 (400 RI)	5 miles at 8:46 ***8km at 5:27***	20 miles at 9:16 ***32km at 5:46***
5	3 x 1600 in 7:19 (400 RI)	10 miles at 8:46 ***16km at 5:27***	15 miles at 9:01 ***24km at 5:36***
4	10 x 400 in 1:44 (400 RI)	8 miles at 8:46 ***13km at 5:27***	20 miles at 9:01 ***32km at 5:36***
3	8 x 800 in 3:32 (90 sec RI)	5 miles at 8:07 ***8km at 5:03***	13 miles at 8:46 ***21km at 5:27***
2	5 x 1000 in 4:27 (400 RI)	2 miles (*3km*) Easy 3 miles at 7:52 ***5km at 4:53***	10 miles at 8:46 ***16km at 5:27***
1	6 x 400 in 1:44 (400 RI)	3 miles at 8:46 ***5km at 5:27***	MARATHON 26.2 miles at 8:46 ***42.2km at 5:27***

For Women 50 to 54, You Must Run 3:55 to BQ

Qualifying for Boston is realistic if you can run:

a 5K in 24:10;
a 10K in 50:34; or
a half-marathon in 1:52:00. (Note: The half-marathon is the best predictor.)

If you can, complete one of each of the three Key Runs in the same week:

Key Run #1: Track repeats (complete one of the workouts listed below)
6 x 800m @ 3:37/800m with a 400m recovery jog between intervals
5 x 1000m @ 4:34 1000m with a 400m recovery jog between intervals
4 x 1200m @ 5:32/1200m with a 400m recovery jog between intervals
3 x 1600m @ 7:31/1600m with a 400m recovery jog between intervals

Key Run #2: Tempo run (complete one of the tempo runs)
After a one-mile warm-up, complete a three-mile training run in 24:12 *or*
After a 1.5km warm-up, complete a 5km training run in 25:05

After a one-mile warm-up, complete a five-mile training run in 41:35 *or*
After a 1.5km warm-up, complete an 8km training run in 41:20

After a one-mile warm-up, complete an eight-mile training run in 68:32 *or*
After a 1.5km warm-up, complete a 13km training run in 69:07

Key Run #3: Long run
Complete a 15- to 20-mile run @ 9:23/mile pace *or*
Complete a 24km to 32km run @ 5:49/km pace

3:55 Boston Marathon Training Plan

RI = Rest Interval; which may be a timed rest/recovery interval or a distance that you walk/jog.
Key Run #1 always begins with a 10–20-min warm-up and ends with a 10-min cool-down.
Key Run #2 begins and ends with a one-mile (1.5km) easy run, unless otherwise indicated.
Metric workout equivalents appear in bold italics.

WEEK	KEY RUN #1	KEY RUN #2	KEY RUN #3
16	3 x 1600 in 7:30 (400 RI)	2 miles (*3km*) Easy 2 miles at 8:04 *3km at 5:01* 2 miles (*3km*) Easy	13 miles at 9:27 *21km at 5:53*
15	4 x 800 in 3:37 (2 min RI)	5 miles at 8:57 *8km at 5:34*	15 miles at 9:42 *24km at 6:02*
14	1200 in 5:32 (200 RI) 1000 in 4:34 (200 RI) 800 in 3:37 (200 RI) 600 in 2:42 (200 RI) 400 in 1:47 (200 RI)	5 miles at 8:34 *8km at 5:19*	17 miles at 9:42 *27km at 6:02*
13	5 x 1000 in 4:34 (400 RI)	4 miles at 8:19 *7km at 5:10*	20 miles at 9:57 *32km at 6:11*
12	3 x 1600 in 7:30 (400 RI)	2 miles (*3km*) Easy 3 miles at 8:04 *5km at 5:01*	18 miles at 9:44 *29km at 6:02*
11	2 x 1200 in 5:32 (2 min RI) 4 x 800 in 3:37 (2 min RI)	5 miles at 8:19 *8km at 5:10*	20 miles at 9:42 *32km at 6:02*
10	6 x 800 in 3:37 (90 sec RI)	6 miles at 8:34 *10km at 5:19*	13 miles at 9:12 *21km at 5:43*
9	2 x (6x 400 in 1:47) (90 sec RI) (2 min 30 sec RI between sets)	2 miles (*3km*) Easy 3 miles at 8:04 *5km at 5:01*	18 miles at 9:27 *29km at 5:53*
8	2 x 1600 in 7:30 (60 sec RI) 2 x 800 in 3:37 (60 sec RI)	4 miles at 8:19 *7km at 5:10*	20 miles at 9:27 *32km at 5:53*
7	4 x 1200 in 5:32 (2 min RI) (4 min RI between sets)	10 miles at 8:57 *16km at 5:34*	15 miles at 9:17 *24km at 5:46*
6	1000 in 4:34, 2000 in 9:28, 1000 in 4:34, 1000 in 4:34 (400 RI)	5 miles at 8:57 *8km at 5:34*	20 miles at 9:27 *32km at 5:53*
5	3 x 1600 in 7:30 (400 RI)	10 miles at 8:57 *16km at 5:34*	15 miles at 9:12 *24km at 5:43*
4	10 x 400 in 1:47 (400 RI)	8 miles at 8:57 *13km at 5:34*	20 miles at 9:12 *32km at 5:43*
3	8 x 800 in 3:37 (90 sec RI)	5 miles at 8:19 *8km at 5:10*	13 miles at 8:57 *21km at 5:34*
2	5 x 1000 in 4:34 (400 RI)	2 miles (*3km*) Easy 3 miles at 8:04 *5km at 5:01*	10 miles at 8:57 *16km at 5:34*
1	6 x 400 in 1:47 (400 RI)	3 miles at 8:57 *5km at 5:34*	MARATHON 26.2 miles at 8:57 *42.2km at 5:34*

For Men 65 to 69 and Women 55 to 59, You Must Run 4:05 to BQ

Qualifying for Boston is realistic if you can run:

a 5K in 25:10;
a 10K in 52:39; or
a half-marathon in 1:56:39. (Note: The half-marathon is the best predictor.)

If you can, complete one of each of the three Key Runs in the same week:

Key Run #1: Track repeats (complete one of the workouts listed below)
6 x 800m @ 3:47/800m with a 400m recovery jog between intervals
5 x 1000m @ 4:46/1000m with a 400m recovery jog between intervals
4 x 1200m @ 5:46/1200m with a 400m recovery jog between intervals
3 x 1600m @ 7:50/1600m with a 400m recovery jog between intervals

Key Run #2: Tempo run (complete one of the tempo runs)
After a one-mile warm-up, complete a three-mile training run in 25:09 *or*
After a 1.5km warm-up, complete a 5km training run in 26:05

After a one-mile warm-up, complete a five-mile training run in 43:10 *or*
After a 1.5km warm-up, complete an 8km training run in 42:56

After a one-mile warm-up, complete an eight-mile training run in 71:04 *or*
After a 1.5km warm-up, complete a 13km training run in 71:43

Key Run #3: Long run
Complete a 15- to 20-mile run @ 9:45/mile pace *or*
Complete a 24km to 32km run @ 6:03/km pace

4:05 Boston Marathon Training Plan

RI = Rest Interval; which may be a timed rest/recovery interval or a distance that you walk/jog.
Key Run #1 always begins with a 10–20-min warm-up and ends with a 10-min cool-down.
Key Run #2 begins and ends with a one-mile (1.5km) easy run, unless otherwise indicated.
Metric workout equivalents appear in bold italics.

WEEK	KEY RUN #1	KEY RUN #2	KEY RUN #3
16	3 x 1600 in 7:50 (400 RI)	2 miles (*3km*) Easy 2 miles at 8:23 *3km at 5:13* 2 miles (*3km*) Easy	13 miles at 9:50 *21km at 6:07*
15	4 x 800 in 3:47 (2 min RI)	5 miles at 9:20 *8km at 5:48*	15 miles at 10:05 *24km at 6:16*
14	1200 in 5:46 (200 RI) 1000 in 4:46 (200 RI) 800 in 3:47 (200 RI) 600 in 2:49 (200 RI) 400 in 1:51 (200 RI)	5 miles at 8:53 *8km at 5:31*	17 miles at 10:05 *27km at 6:16*
13	5 x 1000 in 4:46 (400 RI)	4 miles at 8:38 *7km at 5:22*	20 miles at 10:20 *32km at 6:25*
12	3 x 1600 in 7:50 (400 RI)	2 miles (*3km*) Easy 3 miles at 8:23 *5km at 5:13*	18 miles at 10:05 *29km at 6:16*
11	2 x 1200 in 5:46 (2 min RI) 4 x 800 in 3:47 (2 min RI)	5 miles at 8:38 *8km at 5:22*	20 miles at 10:05 *32km at 6:16*
10	6 x 800 in 3:47 (90 sec RI)	6 miles at 8:53 *10km at 5:31*	13 miles at 9:35 *21km at 5:57*
9	2 x (6x 400 in 1:51) (90 sec RI) (2 min 30 sec RI between sets)	2 miles (*3km*) Easy 3 miles at 8:23 *5km at 5:13*	18 miles at 9:50 *29km at 6:07*
8	2 x 1600 in 7:50 (60 sec RI) 2 x 800 in 3:47 (60 sec RI)	4 miles at 8:38 *7km at 5:22*	20 miles at 9:50 *32km at 6:07*
7	4 x 1200 in 5:46 (2 min RI) (4 min RI between sets)	10 miles at 9:20 *16km at 5:48*	15 miles at 9:40 *24km at 6:00*
6	1000 in 4:46, 2000 in 9:52, 1000 in 4:46, 1000 in 4:46 (400 RI)	5 miles at 9:20 *8km at 5:48*	20 miles at 9:50 *32km at 6:07*
5	3 x 1600 in 7:50 (400 RI)	10 miles at 9:20 *16km at 5:48*	15 miles at 9:35 *24km at 5:57*
4	10 x 400 in 1:51 (400 RI)	8 miles at 9:20 *13km at 5:48*	20 miles at 9:35 *32km at 5:57*
3	8 x 800 in 3:47 (90 sec RI)	5 miles at 8:38 *8km at 5:22*	13 miles at 9:20 *21km at 5:48*
2	5 x 1000 in 4:46 (400 RI)	2 miles (*3km*) Easy 3 miles at 8:23 *5km at 5:13*	10 miles at 9:20 *16km at 5:48*
1	6 x 400 in 1:51 (400 RI)	3 miles at 9:20 *5km at 5:48*	MARATHON 26.2 miles at 9:20 *42.2km at 5:48*

For Men 70 to 74 and Women 60 to 64, You Must Run 4:20 to BQ

Qualifying for Boston is realistic if you can run:

a 5K in 26:43;
a 10K in 55:55; or
a half-marathon in 2:03:51. (Note: The half-marathon is the best predictor.)

If you can, complete one of each of the three Key Runs in the same week:

Key Run #1: Track repeats (complete one of the workouts listed below)
6 x 800m @ 4:02/800m with a 400m recovery jog between intervals
5 x 1000m @ 5:05/1000m with a 400m recovery jog between intervals
4 x 1200m @ 6:09/1200m with a 400m recovery jog between intervals
3 x 1600m @ 8:20/1600m with a 400m recovery jog between intervals

Key Run #2: Tempo run (complete one of the tempo runs)
After a one-mile warm-up, complete a three-mile training run in 26:39 *or*
After a 1.5km warm-up, complete a 5km training run in 27:35

After a one-mile warm-up, complete a five-mile training run in 45:40 *or*
After a 1.5km warm-up, complete an 8km training run in 45:28

After a one-mile warm-up, complete an eight-mile training run in 75:04 *or*
After a 1.5km warm-up, complete a 13km training run in 75:50

Key Run #3: Long run
Complete a 15- to 20-mile run @ 10:20/mile pace *or*
Complete a 24km to 32km run @ 6:26/km pace

4:20 Boston Marathon Training Plan

RI = Rest Interval; which may be a timed rest/recovery interval or a distance that you walk/jog.
Key Run #1 always begins with a 10–20-min warm-up and ends with a 10-min cool-down.
Key Run #2 begins and ends with a one-mile (1.5km) easy run, unless otherwise indicated.
Metric workout equivalents appear in bold italics.

WEEK	KEY RUN #1	KEY RUN #2	KEY RUN #3
16	3 x 1600 in 8:20 (400 RI)	2 miles (**3km**) Easy 2 miles at 8:53 **3km at 5:31** 2 miles (**3km**) Easy	13 miles at 10:25 **21km at 6:28**
15	4 x 800 in 4:02 (2 min RI)	5 miles at 9:55 **8km at 6:09**	15 miles at 10:40 **24km at 6:37**
14	1200 in 6:09 (200 RI) 1000 in 5:05 (200 RI) 800 in 4:02 (200 RI) 600 in 3:00 (200 RI) 400 in 1:59 (200 RI)	5 miles at 9:23 **8km at 5:50**	17 miles at 10:40 **27km at 6:37**
13	5 x 1000 in 5:05 (400 RI)	4 miles at 9:08 **7km at 5:41**	20 miles at 10:55 **32km at 6:46**
12	3 x 1600 in 8:20 (400 RI)	2 miles (**3km**) Easy 3 miles at 8:53 **5km at 5:31**	18 miles at 10:40 **29km at 6:37**
11	2 x 1200 in 6:09 (2 min RI) 4 x 800 in 4:02 (2 min RI)	5 miles at 9:08 **8km at 5:41**	20 miles at 10:40 **32km at 6:37**
10	6 x 800 in 4:02 (90 sec RI)	6 miles at 9:23 **10km at 5:50**	13 miles at 10:10 **21km at 6:18**
9	2 x (6x 400 in 1:59) (90 sec RI) (2 min 30 sec RI between sets)	2 miles (**3km**) Easy 3 miles at 8:53 **5km at 5:31**	18 miles at 10:25 **29km at 6:28**
8	2 x 1600 in 8:20 (60 sec RI) 2 x 800 in 4:02 (60 sec RI)	4 miles at 9:08 **7km at 5:41**	20 miles at 10:25 **32km at 6:28**
7	4 x 1200 in 6:09 (2 min RI) (4 min RI between sets)	10 miles at 9:55 **16km at 6:09**	15 miles at 10:15 **24km at 6:21**
6	1000 in 5:05, 2000 in 10:30, 1000 in 5:05, 1000 in 5:05 (400 RI)	5 miles at 9:55 **8km at 6:09**	20 miles at 10:25 **32km at 6:28**
5	3 x 1600 in 8:20 (400 RI)	10 miles at 9:55 **16km at 6:09**	15 miles at 10:10 **24km at 6:18**
4	10 x 400 in 1:59 (400 RI)	8 miles at 9:55 **13km at 6:09**	20 miles at 10:10 **32km at 6:18**
3	8 x 800 in 4:02 (90 sec RI)	5 miles at 9:08 **8km at 5:41**	13 miles at 9:55 **21km at 6:09**
2	5 x 1000 in 5:05 (400 RI)	2 miles (**3km**) Easy 3 miles at 8:53 **5km at 5:31**	10 miles at 9:55 **16km at 6:09**
1	6 x 400 in 1:59 (400 RI)	3 miles at 9:55 **5km at 6:09**	MARATHON 26.2 miles at 9:55 **42.2km at 6:09**

For Men 75 to 79 and Women 65 to 69, You Must Run 4:35 to BQ

Qualifying for Boston is realistic if you can run:

a 5K in 28:15;
a 10K in 59:05; or
a half-marathon in 2:10:58. (Note: The half-marathon is the best predictor.)

If you can, complete one of each of the three Key Runs in the same week:

Key Run #1: Track repeats (complete one of the workouts listed below)
6 x 800m @ 4:17/800m with a 400m recovery jog between intervals
5 x 1000m @ 5:24/1000m with a 400m recovery jog between intervals
4 x 1200m @ 6:31/1200m with a 400m recovery jog between intervals
3 x 1600m @ 8:50/1600m with a 400m recovery jog between intervals

Key Run #2: Tempo run (complete one of the tempo runs)
After a one-mile warm-up, complete a three-mile training run in 28:09 *or*
After a 1.5km warm-up, complete a 5km training run in 29:10

After a one-mile warm-up, complete a five-mile training run in 48:10 *or*
After a 1.5 kilometer warm-up, complete an 8 kilometer training run in 47:52

After a one-mile warm-up, complete an eight-mile training run in 79:04 *or*
After a 1.5km warm-up, complete a 13km training run in 79:54

Key Run #3: Long run
Complete a 15- to 20-mile run @ 10:54/mile pace *or*
Complete a 24km to 32km run @ 6:47/km pace

4:35 Boston Marathon Training Plan

RI = Rest Interval; which may be a timed rest/recovery interval or a distance that you walk/jog.
Key Run #1 always begins with a 10–20-min warm-up and ends with a 10-min cool-down.
Key Run #2 begins and ends with a one-mile (1.5km) easy run, unless otherwise indicated.
Metric workout equivalents appear in bold italics.

WEEK	KEY RUN #1	KEY RUN #2	KEY RUN #3
16	3 x 1600 in 8:50 (400 RI)	2 miles (***3km***) Easy 2 miles at 9:23 ***3km at 5:49*** 2 miles (***3km***) Easy	13 miles at 10:59 ***21km at 6:50***
15	4 x 800 in 4:17 (2 min RI)	5 miles at 10:29 ***8km at 6:31***	15 miles at 11:14 ***24km at 6:59***
14	1200 in 6:31 (200 RI) 1000 in 5:24 (200 RI) 800 in 4:17 (200 RI) 600 in 3:12 (200 RI) 400 in 2:06 (200 RI)	5 miles at 9:53 ***8km at 6:08***	17 miles at 11:14 ***27km at 6:59***
13	5 x 1000 in 5:24 (400 RI)	4 miles at 9:38 ***7km at 5:59***	20 miles at 11:29 ***32km at 7:08***
12	3 x 1600 in 8:50 (400 RI)	2 miles (***3km***) Easy 3 miles at 9:23 ***5km at 5:49***	18 miles at 11:14 ***29km at 6:59***
11	2 x 1200 in 6:31 (2 min RI) 4 x 800 in 4:17 (2 min RI)	5 miles at 9:38 ***8km at 5:59***	20 miles at 11:14 ***32km at 6:59***
10	6 x 800 in 4:17 (90 sec RI)	6 miles at 9:53 ***10km at 6:08***	13 miles at 10:44 ***21km at 6:40***
9	2 x (6x 400 in 2:06) (90 sec RI) (2 min 30 sec RI between sets)	2 miles (***3km***) Easy 3 miles at 9:23 ***5km at 5:49***	18 miles at 10:59 ***29km at 6:50***
8	2 x 1600 in 8:50 (60 sec RI) 2 x 800 in 4:17 (60 sec RI)	4 miles at 9:38 ***7km at 5:59***	20 miles at 10:59 ***32km at 6:50***
7	4 x 1200 in 6:31 (2 min RI) (4 min RI between sets)	10 miles at 10:29 ***16km at 6:31***	15 miles at 10:49 ***24km at 6:43***
6	1000 in 5:24, 2000 in 11:07, 1000 in 5:24, 1000 in 5:24 (400 RI)	5 miles at 10:29 ***8km at 6:31***	20 miles at 10:59 ***32km at 6:50***
5	3 x 1600 in 8:50 (400 RI)	10 miles at 10:29 ***16km at 6:31***	15 miles at 10:44 ***24km at 6:40***
4	10 x 400 in 2:06 (400 RI)	8 miles at 10:29 ***13km at 6:31***	20 miles at 10:44 ***32km at 6:40***
3	8 x 800 in 4:17 (90 sec RI)	5 miles at 9:38 ***8km at 5:59***	13 miles at 10:29 ***21km at 6:31***
2	5 x 1000 in 5:24 (400 RI)	2 miles (***3km***) Easy 3 miles at 9:23 ***5km at 5:59***	10 miles at 10:29 ***16km at 6:31***
1	6 x 400 in 2:06 (400 RI)	3 miles at 10:29 ***5km at 6:31***	MARATHON 26.2 miles at 10:29 ***42.2km at 6:31***

For Men 80 or Older and Women 70 to 74, You Must Run 4:50 to BQ

Qualifying for Boston is realistic if you can run:

a 5K in 29:49;
a 10K in 62:24; or
a half-marathon in 2:18:15. (Note: The half-marathon is the best predictor.)

If you can, complete one of each of the three Key Runs in the same week:

Key Run #1: Track repeats (complete one of the workouts listed below)
6 x 800m @ 4:32/800m with a 400m recovery jog between intervals
5 x 1000m @ 5:42/1000m with a 400m recovery jog between intervals
4 x 1200m @ 6:54/1200m with a 400m recovery jog between intervals
3 x 1600m @ 9:20/1600m with a 400m recovery jog between intervals

Key Run #2: Tempo run (complete one of the tempo runs)
After a one-mile warm-up, complete a three-mile training run in 29:39 *or*
After a 1.5km warm-up, complete a 5km training run in 30:40

After a one-mile warm-up, complete a five-mile training run in 50:40 *or*
After a 1.5km warm-up, complete an 8km training run in 50:24

After a one-mile warm-up, complete an eight-mile training run in 83:04 *or*
After a 1.5km warm-up, complete a 13km training run in 83:51

Key Run #3: Long run
Complete a 15- to 20-mile run @ 11:29/mile pace *or*
Complete a 24km to 32km run @ 7:09/km pace

4:50 Boston Marathon Training Plan

RI = Rest Interval; which may be a timed rest/recovery interval or a distance that you walk/jog.
Key Run #1 always begins with a 10–20-min warm-up and ends with a 10-min cool-down.
Key Run #2 begins and ends with a one-mile (1.5km) easy run, unless otherwise indicated.
Metric workout equivalents appear in bold italics.

WEEK	KEY RUN #1	KEY RUN #2	KEY RUN #3
16	3 x 1600 in 9:20 (400 RI)	2 miles (*3km*) Easy 2 miles at 9:53 *3km at 6:08* 2 miles (*3km*) Easy	13 miles at 11:33 *21km at 7:11*
15	4 x 800 in 4:32 (2 min RI)	5 miles at 11:03 *8km at 6:52*	15 miles at 11:48 *24km at 7:20*
14	1200 in 6:54 (200 RI) 1000 in 5:42 (200 RI) 800 in 4:32 (200 RI) 600 in 3:23 (200 RI) 400 in 2:14 (200 RI)	5 miles at 10:23 *8km at 6:27*	17 miles at 11:48 *27km at 7:20*
13	5 x 1000 in 5:42 (400 RI)	4 miles at 10:08 *7km at 6:18*	20 miles at 12:03 *32km at 7:29*
12	3 x 1600 in 9:20 (400 RI)	2 miles (*3km*) Easy 3 miles at 9:53 *5km at 6:08*	18 miles at 11:48 *29km at 7:20*
11	2 x 1200 in 6:54 (2 min RI) 4 x 800 in 4:32 (2 min RI)	5 miles at 10:08 *8km at 6:18*	20 miles at 11:48 *32km at 7:20*
10	6 x 800 in 4:32 (90 sec RI)	6 miles at 10:23 *10km at 6:27*	13 miles at 11:18 *21km at 7:01*
9	2 x (6x 400 in 2:14) (90 sec RI) (2 min 30 sec RI between sets)	2 miles (*3km*) Easy 3 miles at 9:53 *5km at 6:08*	18 miles at 11:33 *29km at 7:11*
8	2 x 1600 in 9:20 (60 sec RI) 2 x 800 in 4:32 (60 sec RI)	4 miles at 10:08 *7km at 6:18*	20 miles at 11:33 *32km at 7:11*
7	4 x 1200 in 6:54 (2 min RI) (4 min RI between sets)	10 miles at 11:03 *16km at 6:52*	15 miles at 11:24 *24km at 7:05*
6	1000 in 5:42, 2000 in 11:45, 1000 in 5:42, 1000 in 5:42 (400 RI)	5 miles at 11:03 *8km at 6:52*	20 miles at 11:33 *32km at 7:11*
5	3 x 1600 in 9:20 (400 RI)	10 miles at 11:03 *16km at 6:52*	15 miles at 11:18 *24km at 7:01*
4	10 x 400 in 2:14 (400 RI)	8 miles at 11:03 *13km at 6:52*	20 miles at 11:18 *32km at 7:01*
3	8 x 800 in 4:32 (90 sec RI)	5 miles at 10:08 *8km at 6:18*	13 miles at 11:03 *21km at 6:52*
2	5 x 1000 in 5:42 (400 RI)	2 miles (*3km*) Easy 3 miles at 9:53 *5km at 6:08*	10 miles at 11:03 *16km at 6:52*
1	6 x 400 in 2:14 (400 RI)	3 miles at 11:03 *5km at 6:52*	MARATHON 26.2 miles at 11:03 *42.2km at 6:52*

For Women 75 to 79, You Must Run 5:05 to BQ

Qualifying for Boston is realistic if you can run:

a 5K in 31:20;
a 10K in 65:33; or
a half-marathon in 2:25:14. (Note: The half-marathon is the best predictor.)

If you can, complete one of each of the three Key Runs in the same week:

Key Run #1: Track repeats (complete one of the workouts listed below)
6 x 800m @ 4:47/800m with a 400m recovery jog between intervals
5 x 1000m @ 6:00/1000m with a 400m recovery jog between intervals
4 x 1200m @ 7:16/1200m with a 400m recovery jog between intervals
3 x 1600m @ 9:49/1600m with a 400m recovery jog between intervals

Key Run #2: Tempo run (complete one of the tempo runs)
After a one-mile warm-up, complete a three-mile training run in 31:06 *or*
After a 1.5km warm-up, complete a 5km training run in 32:15

After a one-mile warm-up, complete a five-mile training run in 53:05 *or*
After a 1.5km warm-up, complete an 8km training run in 52:48

After a one-mile warm-up, complete an eight-mile training run in 86:56 *or*
After a 1.5km warm-up, complete a 13km training run in 87:45

Key Run #3: Long run
Complete a 15- to 20-mile run @ 12:03/mile pace *or*
Complete a 24km to 32km run @ 7:30/km pace

5:05 Boston Marathon Training Plan

RI = Rest Interval; which may be a timed rest/recovery interval or a distance that you walk/jog.
Key Run #1 always begins with a 10–20-min warm-up and ends with a 10-min cool-down.
Key Run #2 begins and ends with a one-mile (1.5km) easy run, unless otherwise indicated.
Metric workout equivalents appear in bold italics.

WEEK	KEY RUN #1	KEY RUN #2	KEY RUN #3
16	3 x 1600 in 9:49 (400 RI)	2 miles (*3km*) Easy 2 miles at 10:22 *3km at 6:27* 2 miles (*3km*) Easy	13 miles at 12:08 *21km at 7:32*
15	4 x 800 in 4:47 (2 min RI)	5 miles at 11:38 *8km at 7:13*	15 miles at 12:23 *24km at 7:41*
14	1200 in 7:16 (200 RI) 1000 in 6:00 (200 RI) 800 in 4:47 (200 RI) 600 in 3:34 (200 RI) 400 in 2:21 (200 RI)	5 miles at 10:52 *8km at 6:45*	17 miles at 12:23 *27km at 7:41*
13	5 x 1000 in 6:00 (400 RI)	4 miles at 10:37 *7km at 6:36*	20 miles at 12:38 *32km at 7:50*
12	3 x 1600 in 9:49 (400 RI)	2 miles (*3km*) Easy 3 miles at 10:22 *5km at 6:27*	18 miles at 12:23 *29km at 7:41*
11	2 x 1200 in 7:16 (2 min RI) 4 x 800 in 4:47 (2 min RI)	5 miles at 10:37 *8km at 6:36*	20 miles at 12:23 *32km at 7:41*
10	6 x 800 in 4:47 (90 sec RI)	6 miles at 10:52 *10km at 6:45*	13 miles at 11:53 *21km at 7:22*
9	2 x (6x 400 in 2:21) (90 sec RI) (2 min 30 sec RI between sets)	2 miles (*3km*) Easy 3 miles at 10:22 *5km at 6:27*	18 miles at 12:08 *29km at 7:32*
8	2 x 1600 in 9:49 (60 sec RI) 2 x 800 in 4:47 (60 sec RI)	4 miles at 10:37 *7km at 6:36*	20 miles at 12:08 *32km at 7:32*
7	4 x 1200 in 7:16 (2 min RI) (4 min RI between sets)	10 miles at 11:38 *16km at 7:13*	15 miles at 11:58 *24km at 7:25*
6	1000 in 6:00, 2000 in 12:21, 1000 in 6:00, 1000 in 6:00 (400 RI)	5 miles at 11:38 *8km at 7:13*	20 miles at 12:08 *32km at 7:32*
5	3 x 1600 in 9:49 (400 RI)	10 miles at 11:38 *16km at 7:13*	15 miles at 11:53 *24km at 7:22*
4	10 x 400 in 2:21 (400 RI)	8 miles at 11:38 *13km at 7:13*	20 miles at 11:53 *32km at 7:22*
3	8 x 800 in 4:47 (90 sec RI)	5 miles at 10:37 *8km at 6:36*	13 miles at 11:38 *21km at 7:13*
2	5 x 1000 in 6:00 (400 RI)	2 miles (*3km*) Easy 3 miles at 10:22 *5km at 6:27*	10 miles at 11:38 *16km at 7:13*
1	6 x 400 in 2:21 (400 RI)	3 miles at 11:38 *5km at 7:13*	MARATHON 26.2 miles at 11:38 *42.2km at 7:13*

For Women 80 or Older, You Must Run 5:20 to BQ

Qualifying for Boston is realistic if you can run:

a 5K in 32:53;
a 10K in 1:08:49; or
a half-marathon in 2:32:26. (Note: The half-marathon is the best predictor.)

If you can, complete one of each of the three Key Runs in the same week:

Key Run #1: Track repeats (complete one of the workouts listed below)
6 x 800m @ 5:02/800m with a 400m recovery jog between intervals
5 x 1000m @ 6:19/1000m with a 400m recovery jog between intervals
4 x 1200m @ 7:39/1200m with a 400m recovery jog between intervals
3 x 1600m @ 10:19/1600m with a 400m recovery jog between intervals

Key Run #2: Tempo run (complete one of the tempo runs)
After a one-mile warm-up, complete a three-mile training run in 32:36 *or*
After a 1.5km warm-up, complete a 5km training run in 33:45

After a one-mile warm-up, complete a five-mile training run in 55:35 *or*
After a 1.5km warm-up, complete an 8km training run in 55:20

After a one-mile warm-up, complete an eight-mile training run in 90:56 *or*
After a 1.5km warm-up, complete a 13km training run in 91:52

Key Run #3: Long run
Complete a 15- to 20-mile run @ 12:37/mile pace *or*
Complete a 24km to 32km run @ 7:51/km pace

5:20 Boston Marathon Training Plan

RI = Rest Interval; which may be a timed rest/recovery interval or a distance that you walk/jog.
Key Run #1 always begins with a 10–20-min warm-up and ends with a 10-min cool-down.
Key Run #2 begins and ends with a one-mile (1.5km) easy run, unless otherwise indicated.
Metric workout equivalents appear in bold italics.

WEEK	KEY RUN #1	KEY RUN #2	KEY RUN #3
16	3 x 1600 in 10:19 (400 RI)	2 miles (*3km*) Easy 2 miles at 10:52 ***3km at 6:45*** 2 miles (*3km*) Easy	13 miles at 12:42 ***21km at 7:54***
15	4 x 800 in 5:02 (2 min RI)	5 miles at 12:12 ***8km at 7:35***	15 miles at 12:57 ***24km at 8:03***
14	1200 in 7:39 (200 RI) 1000 in 6:19 (200 RI) 800 in 5:02 (200 RI) 600 in 3:45 (200 RI) 400 in 2:29 (200 RI)	5 miles at 11:22 ***8km at 7:04***	17 miles at 12:57 ***27km at 8:03***
13	5 x 1000 in 6:19 (400 RI)	4 miles at 11:07 ***7km at 6:55***	20 miles at 13:12 ***32km at 8:12***
12	3 x 1600 in 10:19 (400 RI)	2 miles (*3km*) Easy 3 miles at 10:52 ***5km at 6:45***	18 miles at 12:57 ***29km at 8:03***
11	2 x 1200 in 7:39 (2 min RI) 4 x 800 in 5:02 (2 min RI)	5 miles at 11:07 ***8km at 6:55***	20 miles at 12:57 ***32km at 8:03***
10	6 x 800 in 5:02 (90 sec RI)	6 miles at 11:22 ***10km at 7:04***	13 miles at 12:27 ***21km at 7:44***
9	2 x (6x 400 in 2:29) (90 sec RI) (2 min 30 sec RI between sets)	2 miles (*3km*) Easy 3 miles at 10:52 ***5km at 6:45***	18 miles at 12:42 ***29km at 7:54***
8	2 x 1600 in 10:19 (60 sec RI) 2 x 800 in 5:02 (60 sec RI)	4 miles at 11:07 ***7km at 6:55***	20 miles at 12:42 ***32km at 7:54***
7	4 x 1200 in 7:39 (2 min RI) (4 min RI between sets)	10 miles at 12:12 ***16km at 7:35***	15 miles at 12:32 ***24km at 7:47***
6	1000 in 6:19, 2000 in 12:59, 1000 in 6:19, 1000 in 6:19 (400 RI)	5 miles at 12:12 ***8km at 7:35***	20 miles at 12:42 ***32km at 7:54***
5	3 x 1600 in 10:19 (400 RI)	10 miles at 12:12 ***16km at 7:35***	15 miles at 12:27 ***24km at 7:44***
4	10 x 400 in 2:29 (400 RI)	8 miles at 12:12 ***13km at 7:35***	20 miles at 12:27 ***32km at 7:44***
3	8 x 800 in 5:02 (90 sec RI)	5 miles at 11:07 ***8km at 6:55***	13 miles at 12:12 ***21km at 7:35***
2	5 x 1000 in 6:19 (400 RI)	2 miles (*3km*) Easy 3 miles at 10:52 ***5km at 6:45***	10 miles at 12:12 ***16km at 7:35***
1	6 x 400 in 2:29 (400 RI)	3 miles at 12:12 ***5km at 7:35***	MARATHON 26.2 miles at 12:12 ***42.2km at 7:35***

HOW TO CALCULATE PACES

Runners' lives are complicated by the intersection of metric and English race distances and a Babylonian-era base-60 time system. Use these methods to simplify calculating your average race pace.

Changing race time into pace in minutes and seconds per mile:

Take your race time and convert it to total seconds. How? Multiply the number of hours (if any) by 3600. Multiply minutes by 60. Add these two figures and then add the race time seconds to that total. Examples: A marathon run in 3:47:23 equals 10,800 (3 x 3600) + 2,820 (47 x 60) + 23 = 13,643 seconds. A five-mile race run in 33:15 = 1980 (33 x 60) + 15 = 1995 seconds.

Divide the total number of seconds by the distance for the race in miles. If the race is a metric distance, you must find the mile equivalent for the distance. (See the chart below.) Examples from above: Marathon pace = 13,643 seconds / 26.22 miles = 520.3 seconds per mile. Five-mile pace = 1995 seconds / 5 miles = 399 seconds per mile.

Convert the seconds-per-mile pace to minutes and seconds per mile by dividing by 60 and noting the remainder seconds. For the marathon pace:

520.3 seconds per mile / 60 = 8 minutes 40.3 seconds per mile. For the five-mile pace: 399 seconds per mile / 60 = 6 minutes 39 seconds per mile.

Changing race time into pace in minutes and seconds per kilometer:

Take your race time and convert it to total seconds. How? Multiply the number of hours (if any) by 3600. Multiply minutes by 60. Add these two figures and then add the race time seconds to that total. Examples: A marathon run in 3:47:23 equals 10,800 (3 x 3600) + 2,820 (47 x 60) + 23 = 13,643 seconds. An 8km race run in 33:15 = 1980 (33 x 60) + 15 = 1995 seconds.

Divide the total number of seconds by the distance for the race in kilometers. If the race is an imperial distance, you must find the metric equivalent for the distance. (See the chart below.) Examples from above: Marathon pace = 13,643 seconds / 42.2 kilometers = 323.3 seconds per kilometer. 8km pace = 1995 seconds / 8 kilometers = 249.4 seconds per kilometer.

Convert the seconds per kilometer pace to minutes and seconds per kilometer by dividing by 60 and noting the remainder seconds. For the marathon pace: 323.3 seconds per kilometer / 60 = 5 minutes 23.3 seconds per kilometer. For the 8km pace: 249.4 seconds per kilometer / 60 = 4 minutes 9.4 seconds per kilometer.

DISTANCE EQUIVALENTS FOR COMMON RACE DISTANCES

MILES	KILOMETERS	KILOMETERS	MILES
1	1.609	1	.6214
5	8.045	5	3.107
8	12.872	8	4.971
10	16.090	10	6.214
Half-Marathon (13.109)	21.095	15	9.321
15	24.135	20	12.427
20	32.180	Half-Marathon (21.095)	13.109
Marathon (26.219)	42.190	Marathon (42.190)	26.219

RACE TIMES FOR A GIVEN PACE PER MILE

MM:SS/MI	5K	10K	HALF-MARATHON	MARATHON
5:00	15:32	31:05	1:05:33	2:11:06
5:01	15:35	31:11	1:05:46	2:11:32
5:02	15:38	31:17	1:05:59	2:11:58
5:03	15:42	31:23	1:06:12	2:12:24
5:04	15:45	31:29	1:06:25	2:12:51
5:05	15:48	31:36	1:06:38	2:13:17
5:06	15:51	31:42	1:06:51	2:13:43
5:07	15:54	31:48	1:07:05	2:14:09
5:08	15:57	31:54	1:07:18	2:14:35
5:09	16:00	32:00	1:07:31	2:15:02
5:10	16:03	32:07	1:07:44	2:15:28
5:11	16:06	32:13	1:07:57	2:15:54
5:12	16:10	32:19	1:08:10	2:16:20
5:13	16:13	32:25	1:08:23	2:16:46
5:14	16:16	32:32	1:08:36	2:17:13
5:15	16:19	32:38	1:08:49	2:17:39
5:16	16:22	32:44	1:09:03	2:18:05
5:17	16:25	32:50	1:09:16	2:18:31

MM:SS/MI	5K	10K	HALF-MARATHON	MARATHON
5:18	16:28	32:56	1:09:29	2:18:58
5:19	16:31	33:03	1:09:42	2:19:24
5:20	16:34	33:09	1:09:55	2:19:50
5:21	16:38	33:15	1:10:08	2:20:16
5:22	16:41	33:21	1:10:21	2:20:42
5:23	16:44	33:27	1:10:34	2:21:09
5:24	16:47	33:34	1:10:47	2:21:35
5:25	16:50	33:40	1:11:01	2:22:01
5:26	16:53	33:46	1:11:14	2:22:27
5:27	16:56	33:52	1:11:27	2:22:54
5:28	16:59	33:59	1:11:40	2:23:20
5:29	17:02	34:05	1:11:53	2:23:46
5:30	17:05	34:11	1:12:06	2:24:12
5:31	17:09	34:17	1:12:19	2:24:38
5:32	17:12	34:23	1:12:32	2:25:05
5:33	17:15	34:30	1:12:45	2:25:31
5:34	17:18	34:36	1:12:59	2:25:57
5:35	17:21	34:42	1:13:12	2:26:23
5:36	17:24	34:48	1:13:25	2:26:50
5:37	17:27	34:54	1:13:38	2:27:16
5:38	17:30	35:01	1:13:51	2:27:42
5:39	17:33	35:07	1:14:04	2:28:08
5:40	17:37	35:13	1:14:17	2:28:34
5:41	17:40	35:19	1:14:30	2:29:01
5:42	17:43	35:26	1:14:43	2:29:27
5:43	17:46	35:32	1:14:57	2:29:53

MM:SS/MI	5K	10K	HALF-MARATHON	MARATHON
5:44	17:49	35:38	1:15:10	2:30:19
5:45	17:52	35:44	1:15:23	2:30:45
5:46	17:55	35:50	1:15:36	2:31:12
5:47	17:58	35:57	1:15:49	2:31:38
5:48	18:01	36:03	1:16:02	2:32:04
5:49	18:05	36:09	1:16:15	2:32:30
5:50	18:08	36:15	1:16:28	2:32:57
5:51	18:11	36:21	1:16:41	2:33:23
5:52	18:14	36:28	1:16:54	2:33:49
5:53	18:17	36:34	1:17:08	2:34:15
5:54	18:20	36:40	1:17:21	2:34:41
5:55	18:23	36:46	1:17:34	2:35:08
5:56	18:26	36:53	1:17:47	2:35:34
5:57	18:29	36:59	1:18:00	2:36:00
5:58	18:32	37:05	1:18:13	2:36:26
5:59	18:36	37:11	1:18:26	2:36:53
6:00	18:39	37:17	1:18:39	2:37:19
6:01	18:42	37:24	1:18:52	2:37:45
6:02	18:45	37:30	1:19:06	2:38:11
6:03	18:48	37:36	1:19:19	2:38:37
6:04	18:51	37:42	1:19:32	2:39:04
6:05	18:54	37:48	1:19:45	2:39:30
6:06	18:57	37:55	1:19:58	2:39:56
6:07	19:00	38:01	1:20:11	2:40:22
6:08	19:04	38:07	1:20:24	2:40:48
6:09	19:07	38:13	1:20:37	2:41:15

MM:SS/MI	5K	10K	HALF-MARATHON	MARATHON
6:10	19:10	38:20	1:20:50	2:41:41
6:11	19:13	38:26	1:21:04	2:42:07
6:12	19:16	38:32	1:21:17	2:42:33
6:13	19:19	38:38	1:21:30	2:43:00
6:14	19:22	38:44	1:21:43	2:43:26
6:15	19:25	38:51	1:21:56	2:43:52
6:16	19:28	38:57	1:22:09	2:44:18
6:17	19:32	39:03	1:22:22	2:44:44
6:18	19:35	39:09	1:22:35	2:45:11
6:19	19:38	39:16	1:22:48	2:45:37
6:20	19:41	39:22	1:23:02	2:46:03
6:21	19:44	39:28	1:23:15	2:46:29
6:22	19:47	39:34	1:23:28	2:46:56
6:23	19:50	39:40	1:23:41	2:47:22
6:24	19:53	39:47	1:23:54	2:47:48
6:25	19:56	39:53	1:24:07	2:48:14
6:26	20:00	39:59	1:24:20	2:48:40
6:27	20:03	40:05	1:24:33	2:49:07
6:28	20:06	40:11	1:24:46	2:49:33
6:29	20:09	40:18	1:25:00	2:49:59
6:30	20:12	40:24	1:25:13	2:50:25
6:31	20:15	40:30	1:25:26	2:50:52
6:32	20:18	40:36	1:25:39	2:51:18
6:33	20:21	40:43	1:25:52	2:51:44
6:34	20:24	40:49	1:26:05	2:52:10
6:35	20:27	40:55	1:26:18	2:52:36

MM:SS/MI	5K	10K	HALF-MARATHON	MARATHON
6:36	20:31	41:01	1:26:31	2:53:03
6:37	20:34	41:07	1:26:44	2:53:29
6:38	20:37	41:14	1:26:58	2:53:55
6:39	20:40	41:20	1:27:11	2:54:21
6:40	20:43	41:26	1:27:24	2:54:47
6:41	20:46	41:32	1:27:37	2:55:14
6:42	20:49	41:38	1:27:50	2:55:40
6:43	20:52	41:45	1:28:03	2:56:06
6:44	20:55	41:51	1:28:16	2:56:32
6:45	20:59	41:57	1:28:29	2:56:59
6:46	21:02	42:03	1:28:42	2:57:25
6:47	21:05	42:10	1:28:56	2:57:51
6:48	21:08	42:16	1:29:09	2:58:17
6:49	21:11	42:22	1:29:22	2:58:43
6:50	21:14	42:28	1:29:35	2:59:10
6:51	21:17	42:34	1:29:48	2:59:36
6:52	21:20	42:41	1:30:01	3:00:02
6:53	21:23	42:47	1:30:14	3:00:28
6:54	21:27	42:53	1:30:27	3:00:55
6:55	21:30	42:59	1:30:40	3:01:21
6:56	21:33	43:05	1:30:53	3:01:47
6:57	21:36	43:12	1:31:07	3:02:13
6:58	21:39	43:18	1:31:20	3:02:39
6:59	21:42	43:24	1:31:33	3:03:06
7:00	21:45	43:30	1:31:46	3:03:32
7:01	21:48	43:37	1:31:59	3:03:58

MM:SS/MI	5K	10K	HALF-MARATHON	MARATHON
7:02	21:51	43:43	1:32:12	3:04:24
7:03	21:54	43:49	1:32:25	3:04:51
7:04	21:58	43:55	1:32:38	3:05:17
7:05	22:01	44:01	1:32:51	3:05:43
7:06	22:04	44:08	1:33:05	3:06:09
7:07	22:07	44:14	1:33:18	3:06:35
7:08	22:10	44:20	1:33:31	3:07:02
7:09	22:13	44:26	1:33:44	3:07:28
7:10	22:16	44:32	1:33:57	3:07:54
7:11	22:19	44:39	1:34:10	3:08:20
7:12	22:22	44:45	1:34:23	3:08:46
7:13	22:26	44:51	1:34:36	3:09:13
7:14	22:29	44:57	1:34:49	3:09:39
7:15	22:32	45:04	1:35:03	3:10:05
7:16	22:35	45:10	1:35:16	3:10:31
7:17	22:38	45:16	1:35:29	3:10:58
7:18	22:41	45:22	1:35:42	3:11:24
7:19	22:44	45:28	1:35:55	3:11:50
7:20	22:47	45:35	1:36:08	3:12:16
7:21	22:50	45:41	1:36:21	3:12:42
7:22	22:54	45:47	1:36:34	3:13:09
7:23	22:57	45:53	1:36:47	3:13:35
7:24	23:00	45:59	1:37:01	3:14:01
7:25	23:03	46:06	1:37:14	3:14:27
7:26	23:06	46:12	1:37:27	3:14:54
7:27	23:09	46:18	1:37:40	3:15:20

MM:SS/MI	5K	10K	HALF-MARATHON	MARATHON
7:28	23:12	46:24	1:37:53	3:15:46
7:29	23:15	46:31	1:38:06	3:16:12
7:30	23:18	46:37	1:38:19	3:16:38
7:31	23:21	46:43	1:38:32	3:17:05
7:32	23:25	46:49	1:38:45	3:17:31
7:33	23:28	46:55	1:38:59	3:17:57
7:34	23:31	47:02	1:39:12	3:18:23
7:35	23:34	47:08	1:39:25	3:18:50
7:36	23:37	47:14	1:39:38	3:19:16
7:37	23:40	47:20	1:39:51	3:19:42
7:38	23:43	47:26	1:40:04	3:20:08
7:39	23:46	47:33	1:40:17	3:20:34
7:40	23:49	47:39	1:40:30	3:21:01
7:41	23:53	47:45	1:40:43	3:21:27
7:42	23:56	47:51	1:40:57	3:21:53
7:43	23:59	47:58	1:41:10	3:22:19
7:44	24:02	48:04	1:41:23	3:22:45
7:45	24:05	48:10	1:41:36	3:23:12
7:46	24:08	48:16	1:41:49	3:23:38
7:47	24:11	48:22	1:42:02	3:24:04
7:48	24:14	48:29	1:42:15	3:24:30
7:49	24:17	48:35	1:42:28	3:24:57
7:50	24:21	48:41	1:42:41	3:25:23
7:51	24:24	48:47	1:42:55	3:25:49
7:52	24:27	48:53	1:43:08	3:26:15
7:53	24:30	49:00	1:43:21	3:26:41

MM:SS/MI	5K	10K	HALF-MARATHON	MARATHON
7:54	24:33	49:06	1:43:34	3:27:08
7:55	24:36	49:12	1:43:47	3:27:34
7:56	24:39	49:18	1:44:00	3:28:00
7:57	24:42	49:25	1:44:13	3:28:26
7:58	24:45	49:31	1:44:26	3:28:53
7:59	24:49	49:37	1:44:39	3:29:19
8:00	24:52	49:43	1:44:52	3:29:45
8:01	24:55	49:49	1:45:06	3:30:11
8:02	24:58	49:56	1:45:19	3:30:37
8:03	25:01	50:02	1:45:32	3:31:04
8:04	25:04	50:08	1:45:45	3:31:30
8:05	25:07	50:14	1:45:58	3:31:56
8:06	25:10	50:21	1:46:11	3:32:22
8:07	25:13	50:27	1:46:24	3:32:49
8:08	25:16	50:33	1:46:37	3:33:15
8:09	25:20	50:39	1:46:50	3:33:41
8:10	25:23	50:45	1:47:04	3:34:07
8:11	25:26	50:52	1:47:17	3:34:33
8:12	25:29	50:58	1:47:30	3:35:00
8:13	25:32	51:04	1:47:43	3:35:26
8:14	25:35	51:10	1:47:56	3:35:52
8:15	25:38	51:16	1:48:09	3:36:18
8:16	25:41	51:23	1:48:22	3:36:44
8:17	25:44	51:29	1:48:35	3:37:11
8:18	25:48	51:35	1:48:48	3:37:37
8:19	25:51	51:41	1:49:02	3:38:03

MM:SS/MI	5K	10K	HALF-MARATHON	MARATHON
8:20	25:54	51:48	1:49:15	3:38:29
8:21	25:57	51:54	1:49:28	3:38:56
8:22	26:00	52:00	1:49:41	3:39:22
8:23	26:03	52:06	1:49:54	3:39:48
8:24	26:06	52:12	1:50:07	3:40:14
8:25	26:09	52:19	1:50:20	3:40:40
8:26	26:12	52:25	1:50:33	3:41:07
8:27	26:16	52:31	1:50:46	3:41:33
8:28	26:19	52:37	1:51:00	3:41:59
8:29	26:22	52:43	1:51:13	3:42:25
8:30	26:25	52:50	1:51:26	3:42:52
8:31	26:28	52:56	1:51:39	3:43:18
8:32	26:31	53:02	1:51:52	3:43:44
8:33	26:34	53:08	1:52:05	3:44:10
8:34	26:37	53:15	1:52:18	3:44:36
8:35	26:40	53:21	1:52:31	3:45:03
8:36	26:43	53:27	1:52:44	3:45:29
8:37	26:47	53:33	1:52:58	3:45:55
8:38	26:50	53:39	1:53:11	3:46:21
8:39	26:53	53:46	1:53:24	3:46:48
8:40	26:56	53:52	1:53:37	3:47:14
8:41	26:59	53:58	1:53:50	3:47:40
8:42	27:02	54:04	1:54:03	3:48:06
8:43	27:05	54:10	1:54:16	3:48:32
8:44	27:08	54:17	1:54:29	3:48:59
8:45	27:11	54:23	1:54:42	3:49:25

MM:SS/MI	5K	10K	HALF-MARATHON	MARATHON
8:46	27:15	54:29	1:54:56	3:49:51
8:47	27:18	54:35	1:55:09	3:50:17
8:48	27:21	54:42	1:55:22	3:50:43
8:49	27:24	54:48	1:55:35	3:51:10
8:50	27:27	54:54	1:55:48	3:51:36
8:51	27:30	55:00	1:56:01	3:52:02
8:52	27:33	55:06	1:56:14	3:52:28
8:53	27:36	55:13	1:56:27	3:52:55
8:54	27:39	55:19	1:56:40	3:53:21
8:55	27:43	55:25	1:56:54	3:53:47
8:56	27:46	55:31	1:57:07	3:54:13
8:57	27:49	55:37	1:57:20	3:54:39
8:58	27:52	55:44	1:57:33	3:55:06
8:59	27:55	55:50	1:57:46	3:55:32
9:00	27:58	55:56	1:57:59	3:55:58
9:01	28:01	56:02	1:58:12	3:56:24
9:02	28:04	56:09	1:58:25	3:56:51
9:03	28:07	56:15	1:58:38	3:57:17
9:04	28:10	56:21	1:58:51	3:57:43
9:05	28:14	56:27	1:59:05	3:58:09
9:06	28:17	56:33	1:59:18	3:58:35
9:07	28:20	56:40	1:59:31	3:59:02
9:08	28:23	56:46	1:59:44	3:59:28
9:09	28:26	56:52	1:59:57	3:59:54
9:10	28:29	56:58	2:00:10	4:00:20
9:11	28:32	57:04	2:00:23	4:00:47

MM:SS/MI	5K	10K	HALF-MARATHON	MARATHON
9:12	28:35	57:11	2:00:36	4:01:13
9:13	28:38	57:17	2:00:49	4:01:39
9:14	28:42	57:23	2:01:03	4:02:05
9:15	28:45	57:29	2:01:16	4:02:31
9:16	28:48	57:36	2:01:29	4:02:58
9:17	28:51	57:42	2:01:42	4:03:24
9:18	28:54	57:48	2:01:55	4:03:50
9:19	28:57	57:54	2:02:08	4:04:16
9:20	29:00	58:00	2:02:21	4:04:42
9:21	29:03	58:07	2:02:34	4:05:09
9:22	29:06	58:13	2:02:47	4:05:35
9:23	29:10	58:19	2:03:01	4:06:01
9:24	29:13	58:25	2:03:14	4:06:27
9:25	29:16	58:31	2:03:27	4:06:54
9:26	29:19	58:38	2:03:40	4:07:20
9:27	29:22	58:44	2:03:53	4:07:46
9:28	29:25	58:50	2:04:06	4:08:12
9:29	29:28	58:56	2:04:19	4:08:38
9:30	29:31	59:03	2:04:32	4:09:05
9:31	29:34	59:09	2:04:45	4:09:31
9:32	29:38	59:15	2:04:59	4:09:57
9:33	29:41	59:21	2:05:12	4:10:23
9:34	29:44	59:27	2:05:25	4:10:50
9:35	29:47	59:34	2:05:38	4:11:16
9:36	29:50	59:40	2:05:51	4:11:42
9:37	29:53	59:46	2:06:04	4:12:08

MM:SS/MI	5K	10K	HALF-MARATHON	MARATHON
9:38	29:56	59:52	2:06:17	4:12:34
9:39	29:59	59:59	2:06:30	4:13:01
9:40	30:02	1:00:05	2:06:43	4:13:27
9:41	30:05	1:00:11	2:06:57	4:13:53
9:42	30:09	1:00:17	2:07:10	4:14:19
9:43	30:12	1:00:23	2:07:23	4:14:46
9:44	30:15	1:00:30	2:07:36	4:15:12
9:45	30:18	1:00:36	2:07:49	4:15:38
9:46	30:21	1:00:42	2:08:02	4:16:04
9:47	30:24	1:00:48	2:08:15	4:16:30
9:48	30:27	1:00:54	2:08:28	4:16:57
9:49	30:30	1:01:01	2:08:41	4:17:23
9:50	30:33	1:01:07	2:08:55	4:17:49
9:51	30:37	1:01:13	2:09:08	4:18:15
9:52	30:40	1:01:19	2:09:21	4:18:41
9:53	30:43	1:01:26	2:09:34	4:19:08
9:54	30:46	1:01:32	2:09:47	4:19:34
9:55	30:49	1:01:38	2:10:00	4:20:00
9:56	30:52	1:01:44	2:10:13	4:20:26
9:57	30:55	1:01:50	2:10:26	4:20:53
9:58	30:58	1:01:57	2:10:39	4:21:19
9:59	31:01	1:02:03	2:10:53	4:21:45
10:00	31:05	1:02:09	2:11:06	4:22:11
10:01	31:08	1:02:15	2:11:19	4:22:37
10:02	31:11	1:02:21	2:11:32	4:23:04
10:03	31:14	1:02:28	2:11:45	4:23:30

MM:SS/MI	5K	10K	HALF-MARATHON	MARATHON
10:04	31:17	1:02:34	2:11:58	4:23:56
10:05	31:20	1:02:40	2:12:11	4:24:22
10:06	31:23	1:02:46	2:12:24	4:24:49
10:07	31:26	1:02:53	2:12:37	4:25:15
10:08	31:29	1:02:59	2:12:50	4:25:41
10:09	31:32	1:03:05	2:13:04	4:26:07
10:10	31:36	1:03:11	2:13:17	4:26:33
10:11	31:39	1:03:17	2:13:30	4:27:00
10:12	31:42	1:03:24	2:13:43	4:27:26
10:13	31:45	1:03:30	2:13:56	4:27:52
10:14	31:48	1:03:36	2:14:09	4:28:18
10:15	31:51	1:03:42	2:14:22	4:28:45
10:16	31:54	1:03:48	2:14:35	4:29:11
10:17	31:57	1:03:55	2:14:48	4:29:37
10:18	32:00	1:04:01	2:15:02	4:30:03
10:19	32:04	1:04:07	2:15:15	4:30:29
10:20	32:07	1:04:13	2:15:28	4:30:56
10:21	32:10	1:04:20	2:15:41	4:31:22
10:22	32:13	1:04:26	2:15:54	4:31:48
10:23	32:16	1:04:32	2:16:07	4:32:14
10:24	32:19	1:04:38	2:16:20	4:32:40
10:25	32:22	1:04:44	2:16:33	4:33:07
10:26	32:25	1:04:51	2:16:46	4:33:33
10:27	32:28	1:04:57	2:17:00	4:33:59
10:28	32:32	1:05:03	2:17:13	4:34:25
10:29	32:35	1:05:09	2:17:26	4:34:52

MM:SS/MI	5K	10K	HALF-MARATHON	MARATHON
10:30	32:38	1:05:15	2:17:39	4:35:18
10:31	32:41	1:05:22	2:17:52	4:35:44
10:32	32:44	1:05:28	2:18:05	4:36:10
10:33	32:47	1:05:34	2:18:18	4:36:36
10:34	32:50	1:05:40	2:18:31	4:37:03
10:35	32:53	1:05:47	2:18:44	4:37:29
10:36	32:56	1:05:53	2:18:58	4:37:55
10:37	32:59	1:05:59	2:19:11	4:38:21
10:38	33:03	1:06:05	2:19:24	4:38:48
10:39	33:06	1:06:11	2:19:37	4:39:14
10:40	33:09	1:06:18	2:19:50	4:39:40
10:41	33:12	1:06:24	2:20:03	4:40:06
10:42	33:15	1:06:30	2:20:16	4:40:32
10:43	33:18	1:06:36	2:20:29	4:40:59
10:44	33:21	1:06:42	2:20:42	4:41:25
10:45	33:24	1:06:49	2:20:56	4:41:51
10:46	33:27	1:06:55	2:21:09	4:42:17
10:47	33:31	1:07:01	2:21:22	4:42:44
10:48	33:34	1:07:07	2:21:35	4:43:10
10:49	33:37	1:07:14	2:21:48	4:43:36
10:50	33:40	1:07:20	2:22:01	4:44:02
10:51	33:43	1:07:26	2:22:14	4:44:28
10:52	33:46	1:07:32	2:22:27	4:44:55
10:53	33:49	1:07:38	2:22:40	4:45:21
10:54	33:52	1:07:45	2:22:54	4:45:47
10:55	33:55	1:07:51	2:23:07	4:46:13

MM:SS/MI	5K	10K	HALF-MARATHON	MARATHON
10:56	33:59	1:07:57	2:23:20	4:46:39
10:57	34:02	1:08:03	2:23:33	4:47:06
10:58	34:05	1:08:09	2:23:46	4:47:32
10:59	34:08	1:08:16	2:23:59	4:47:58
11:00	34:11	1:08:22	2:24:12	4:48:24
11:01	34:14	1:08:28	2:24:25	4:48:51
11:02	34:17	1:08:34	2:24:38	4:49:17
11:03	34:20	1:08:41	2:24:52	4:49:43
11:04	34:23	1:08:47	2:25:05	4:50:09
11:05	34:27	1:08:53	2:25:18	4:50:35
11:06	34:30	1:08:59	2:25:31	4:51:02
11:07	34:33	1:09:05	2:25:44	4:51:28
11:08	34:36	1:09:12	2:25:57	4:51:54
11:09	34:39	1:09:18	2:26:10	4:52:20
11:10	34:42	1:09:24	2:26:23	4:52:47
11:11	34:45	1:09:30	2:26:36	4:53:13
11:12	34:48	1:09:37	2:26:49	4:53:39
11:13	34:51	1:09:43	2:27:03	4:54:05
11:14	34:54	1:09:49	2:27:16	4:54:31
11:15	34:58	1:09:55	2:27:29	4:54:58
11:16	35:01	1:10:01	2:27:42	4:55:24
11:17	35:04	1:10:08	2:27:55	4:55:50
11:18	35:07	1:10:14	2:28:08	4:56:16
11:19	35:10	1:10:20	2:28:21	4:56:43
11:20	35:13	1:10:26	2:28:34	4:57:09
11:21	35:16	1:10:32	2:28:47	4:57:35

MM:SS/MI	5K	10K	HALF-MARATHON	MARATHON
11:22	35:19	1:10:39	2:29:01	4:58:01
11:23	35:22	1:10:45	2:29:14	4:58:27
11:24	35:26	1:10:51	2:29:27	4:58:54
11:25	35:29	1:10:57	2:29:40	4:59:20
11:26	35:32	1:11:04	2:29:53	4:59:46
11:27	35:35	1:11:10	2:30:06	5:00:12
11:28	35:38	1:11:16	2:30:19	5:00:38
11:29	35:41	1:11:22	2:30:32	5:01:05
11:30	35:44	1:11:28	2:30:45	5:01:31
11:31	35:47	1:11:35	2:30:59	5:01:57
11:32	35:50	1:11:41	2:31:12	5:02:23
11:33	35:54	1:11:47	2:31:25	5:02:50
11:34	35:57	1:11:53	2:31:38	5:03:16
11:35	36:00	1:11:59	2:31:51	5:03:42
11:36	36:03	1:12:06	2:32:04	5:04:08
11:37	36:06	1:12:12	2:32:17	5:04:34
11:38	36:09	1:12:18	2:32:30	5:05:01
11:39	36:12	1:12:24	2:32:43	5:05:27
11:40	36:15	1:12:31	2:32:57	5:05:53
11:41	36:18	1:12:37	2:33:10	5:06:19
11:42	36:21	1:12:43	2:33:23	5:06:46
11:43	36:25	1:12:49	2:33:36	5:07:12
11:44	36:28	1:12:55	2:33:49	5:07:38
11:45	36:31	1:13:02	2:34:02	5:08:04
11:46	36:34	1:13:08	2:34:15	5:08:30
11:47	36:37	1:13:14	2:34:28	5:08:57

MM:SS/MI	5K	10K	HALF-MARATHON	MARATHON
11:48	36:40	1:13:20	2:34:41	5:09:23
11:49	36:43	1:13:26	2:34:55	5:09:49
11:50	36:46	1:13:33	2:35:08	5:10:15
11:51	36:49	1:13:39	2:35:21	5:10:42
11:52	36:53	1:13:45	2:35:34	5:11:08
11:53	36:56	1:13:51	2:35:47	5:11:34
11:54	36:59	1:13:58	2:36:00	5:12:00
11:55	37:02	1:14:04	2:36:13	5:12:26
11:56	37:05	1:14:10	2:36:26	5:12:53
11:57	37:08	1:14:16	2:36:39	5:13:19
11:58	37:11	1:14:22	2:36:53	5:13:45
11:59	37:14	1:14:29	2:37:06	5:14:11
12:00	37:17	1:14:35	2:37:19	5:14:37
12:01	37:21	1:14:41	2:37:32	5:15:04
12:02	37:24	1:14:47	2:37:45	5:15:30
12:03	37:27	1:14:53	2:37:58	5:15:56
12:04	37:30	1:15:00	2:38:11	5:16:22
12:05	37:33	1:15:06	2:38:24	5:16:49
12:06	37:36	1:15:12	2:38:37	5:17:15
12:07	37:39	1:15:18	2:38:51	5:17:41
12:08	37:42	1:15:25	2:39:04	5:18:07
12:09	37:45	1:15:31	2:39:17	5:18:33
12:10	37:48	1:15:37	2:39:30	5:19:00
12:11	37:52	1:15:43	2:39:43	5:19:26
12:12	37:55	1:15:49	2:39:56	5:19:52
12:13	37:58	1:15:56	2:40:09	5:20:18

MM:SS/MI	5K	10K	HALF-MARATHON	MARATHON
12:14	38:01	1:16:02	2:40:22	5:20:45
12:15	38:04	1:16:08	2:40:35	5:21:11
12:16	38:07	1:16:14	2:40:48	5:21:37
12:17	38:10	1:16:20	2:41:02	5:22:03
12:18	38:13	1:16:27	2:41:15	5:22:29
12:19	38:16	1:16:33	2:41:28	5:22:56
12:20	38:20	1:16:39	2:41:41	5:23:22
12:21	38:23	1:16:45	2:41:54	5:23:48
12:22	38:26	1:16:52	2:42:07	5:24:14
12:23	38:29	1:16:58	2:42:20	5:24:41
12:24	38:32	1:17:04	2:42:33	5:25:07
12:25	38:35	1:17:10	2:42:46	5:25:33
12:26	38:38	1:17:16	2:43:00	5:25:59
12:27	38:41	1:17:23	2:43:13	5:26:25
12:28	38:44	1:17:29	2:43:26	5:26:52
12:29	38:48	1:17:35	2:43:39	5:27:18
12:30	38:51	1:17:41	2:43:52	5:27:44
12:31	38:54	1:17:47	2:44:05	5:28:10
12:32	38:57	1:17:54	2:44:18	5:28:36
12:33	39:00	1:18:00	2:44:31	5:29:03
12:34	39:03	1:18:06	2:44:44	5:29:29
12:35	39:06	1:18:12	2:44:58	5:29:55
12:36	39:09	1:18:19	2:45:11	5:30:21
12:37	39:12	1:18:25	2:45:24	5:30:48
12:38	39:16	1:18:31	2:45:37	5:31:14
12:39	39:19	1:18:37	2:45:50	5:31:40

MM:SS/MI	5K	10K	HALF-MARATHON	MARATHON
12:40	39:22	1:18:43	2:46:03	5:32:06
12:41	39:25	1:18:50	2:46:16	5:32:32
12:42	39:28	1:18:56	2:46:29	5:32:59
12:43	39:31	1:19:02	2:46:42	5:33:25
12:44	39:34	1:19:08	2:46:56	5:33:51
12:45	39:37	1:19:15	2:47:09	5:34:17
12:46	39:40	1:19:21	2:47:22	5:34:44
12:47	39:43	1:19:27	2:47:35	5:35:10
12:48	39:47	1:19:33	2:47:48	5:35:36
12:49	39:50	1:19:39	2:48:01	5:36:02
12:50	39:53	1:19:46	2:48:14	5:36:28
12:51	39:56	1:19:52	2:48:27	5:36:55
12:52	39:59	1:19:58	2:48:40	5:37:21
12:53	40:02	1:20:04	2:48:54	5:37:47
12:54	40:05	1:20:10	2:49:07	5:38:13
12:55	40:08	1:20:17	2:49:20	5:38:40
12:56	40:11	1:20:23	2:49:33	5:39:06
12:57	40:15	1:20:29	2:49:46	5:39:32

RACE TIMES FOR A GIVEN PACE PER KILOMETER

MM:SS/MI	5K	10K	HALF-MARATHON	MARATHON
3:06	15:30	31:00	1:05:23	2:10:47
3:07	15:35	31:10	1:05:44	2:11:29
3:08	15:40	31:20	1:06:05	2:12:11
3:09	15:45	31:30	1:06:27	2:12:53
3:10	15:50	31:40	1:06:48	2:13:35
3:11	15:55	31:50	1:07:09	2:14:18
3:12	16:00	32:00	1:07:30	2:15:00
3:13	16:05	32:10	1:07:51	2:15:42
3:14	16:10	32:20	1:08:12	2:16:24
3:15	16:15	32:30	1:08:33	2:17:06
3:16	16:20	32:40	1:08:54	2:17:48
3:17	16:25	32:50	1:09:15	2:18:31
3:18	16:30	33:00	1:09:36	2:19:13
3:19	16:35	33:10	1:09:58	2:19:55
3:20	16:40	33:20	1:10:19	2:20:37
3:21	16:45	33:30	1:10:40	2:21:19
3:22	16:50	33:40	1:11:01	2:22:02
3:23	16:55	33:50	1:11:22	2:22:44
3:24	17:00	34:00	1:11:43	2:23:26
3:25	17:05	34:10	1:12:04	2:24:08
3:26	17:10	34:20	1:12:25	2:24:50
3:27	17:15	34:30	1:12:46	2:25:33
3:28	17:20	34:40	1:13:07	2:26:15
3:29	17:25	34:50	1:13:28	2:26:57

MM:SS/MI	5K	10K	HALF-MARATHON	MARATHON
3:30	17:30	35:00	1:13:50	2:27:39
3:31	17:35	35:10	1:14:11	2:28:21
3:32	17:40	35:20	1:14:32	2:29:03
3:33	17:45	35:30	1:14:53	2:29:46
3:34	17:50	35:40	1:15:14	2:30:28
3:35	17:55	35:50	1:15:35	2:31:10
3:36	18:00	36:00	1:15:56	2:31:52
3:37	18:05	36:10	1:16:17	2:32:34
3:38	18:10	36:20	1:16:38	2:33:17
3:39	18:15	36:30	1:16:59	2:33:59
3:40	18:20	36:40	1:17:20	2:34:41
3:41	18:25	36:50	1:17:42	2:35:23
3:42	18:30	37:00	1:18:03	2:36:05
3:43	18:35	37:10	1:18:24	2:36:47
3:44	18:40	37:20	1:18:45	2:37:30
3:45	18:45	37:30	1:19:06	2:38:12
3:46	18:50	37:40	1:19:27	2:38:54
3:47	18:55	37:50	1:19:48	2:39:36
3:48	19:00	38:00	1:20:09	2:40:18
3:49	19:05	38:10	1:20:30	2:41:01
3:50	19:10	38:20	1:20:51	2:41:43
3:51	19:15	38:30	1:21:12	2:42:25
3:52	19:20	38:40	1:21:34	2:43:07
3:53	19:25	38:50	1:21:55	2:43:49
3:54	19:30	39:00	1:22:16	2:44:32
3:55	19:35	39:10	1:22:37	2:45:14

MM:SS/MI	5K	10K	HALF-MARATHON	MARATHON
3:56	19:40	39:20	1:22:58	2:45:56
3:57	19:45	39:30	1:23:19	2:46:38
3:58	19:50	39:40	1:23:40	2:47:20
3:59	19:55	39:50	1:24:01	2:48:02
4:00	20:00	40:00	1:24:22	2:48:45
4:01	20:05	40:10	1:24:43	2:49:27
4:02	20:10	40:20	1:25:05	2:50:09
4:03	20:15	40:30	1:25:26	2:50:51
4:04	20:20	40:40	1:25:47	2:51:33
4:05	20:25	40:50	1:26:08	2:52:16
4:06	20:30	41:00	1:26:29	2:52:58
4:07	20:35	41:10	1:26:50	2:53:40
4:08	20:40	41:20	1:27:11	2:54:22
4:09	20:45	41:30	1:27:32	2:55:04
4:10	20:50	41:40	1:27:53	2:55:46
4:11	20:55	41:50	1:28:14	2:56:29
4:12	21:00	42:00	1:28:35	2:57:11
4:13	21:05	42:10	1:28:57	2:57:53
4:14	21:10	42:20	1:29:18	2:58:35
4:15	21:15	42:30	1:29:39	2:59:17
4:16	21:20	42:40	1:30:00	3:00:00
4:17	21:25	42:50	1:30:21	3:00:42
4:18	21:30	43:00	1:30:42	3:01:24
4:19	21:35	43:10	1:31:03	3:02:06
4:20	21:40	43:20	1:31:24	3:02:48
4:21	21:45	43:30	1:31:45	3:03:31

MM:SS/MI	5K	10K	HALF-MARATHON	MARATHON
4:22	21:50	43:40	1:32:06	3:04:13
4:23	21:55	43:50	1:32:27	3:04:55
4:24	22:00	44:00	1:32:49	3:05:37
4:25	22:05	44:10	1:33:10	3:06:19
4:26	22:10	44:20	1:33:31	3:07:01
4:27	22:15	44:30	1:33:52	3:07:44
4:28	22:20	44:40	1:34:13	3:08:26
4:29	22:25	44:50	1:34:34	3:09:08
4:30	22:30	45:00	1:34:55	3:09:50
4:31	22:35	45:10	1:35:16	3:10:32
4:32	22:40	45:20	1:35:37	3:11:15
4:33	22:45	45:30	1:35:58	3:11:57
4:34	22:50	45:40	1:36:19	3:12:39
4:35	22:55	45:50	1:36:41	3:13:21
4:36	23:00	46:00	1:37:02	3:14:03
4:37	23:05	46:10	1:37:23	3:14:46
4:38	23:10	46:20	1:37:44	3:15:28
4:39	23:15	46:30	1:38:05	3:16:10
4:40	23:20	46:40	1:38:26	3:16:52
4:41	23:25	46:50	1:38:47	3:17:34
4:42	23:30	47:00	1:39:08	3:18:16
4:43	23:35	47:10	1:39:29	3:18:59
4:44	23:40	47:20	1:39:50	3:19:41
4:45	23:45	47:30	1:40:12	3:20:23
4:46	23:50	47:40	1:40:33	3:21:05
4:47	23:55	47:50	1:40:54	3:21:47

MM:SS/MI	5K	10K	HALF-MARATHON	MARATHON
4:48	24:00	48:00	1:41:15	3:22:30
4:49	24:05	48:10	1:41:36	3:23:12
4:50	24:10	48:20	1:41:57	3:23:54
4:51	24:15	48:30	1:42:18	3:24:36
4:52	24:20	48:40	1:42:39	3:25:18
4:53	24:25	48:50	1:43:00	3:26:00
4:54	24:30	49:00	1:43:21	3:26:43
4:55	24:35	49:10	1:43:42	3:27:25
4:56	24:40	49:20	1:44:04	3:28:07
4:57	24:45	49:30	1:44:25	3:28:49
4:58	24:50	49:40	1:44:46	3:29:31
4:59	24:55	49:50	1:45:07	3:30:14
5:00	25:00	50:00	1:45:28	3:30:56
5:01	25:05	50:10	1:45:49	3:31:38
5:02	25:10	50:20	1:46:10	3:32:20
5:03	25:15	50:30	1:46:31	3:33:02
5:04	25:20	50:40	1:46:52	3:33:45
5:05	25:25	50:50	1:47:13	3:34:27
5:06	25:30	51:00	1:47:34	3:35:09
5:07	25:35	51:10	1:47:56	3:35:51
5:08	25:40	51:20	1:48:17	3:36:33
5:09	25:45	51:30	1:48:38	3:37:15
5:10	25:50	51:40	1:48:59	3:37:58
5:11	25:55	51:50	1:49:20	3:38:40
5:12	26:00	52:00	1:49:41	3:39:22
5:13	26:05	52:10	1:50:02	3:40:04

MM:SS/MI	5K	10K	HALF-MARATHON	MARATHON
5:14	26:10	52:20	1:50:23	3:40:46
5:15	26:15	52:30	1:50:44	3:41:29
5:16	26:20	52:40	1:51:05	3:42:11
5:17	26:25	52:50	1:51:26	3:42:53
5:18	26:30	53:00	1:51:48	3:43:35
5:19	26:35	53:10	1:52:09	3:44:17
5:20	26:40	53:20	1:52:30	3:45:00
5:21	26:45	53:30	1:52:51	3:45:42
5:22	26:50	53:40	1:53:12	3:46:24
5:23	26:55	53:50	1:53:33	3:47:06
5:24	27:00	54:00	1:53:54	3:47:48
5:25	27:05	54:10	1:54:15	3:48:30
5:26	27:10	54:20	1:54:36	3:49:13
5:27	27:15	54:30	1:54:57	3:49:55
5:28	27:20	54:40	1:55:19	3:50:37
5:29	27:25	54:50	1:55:40	3:51:19
5:30	27:30	55:00	1:56:01	3:52:01
5:31	27:35	55:10	1:56:22	3:52:44
5:32	27:40	55:20	1:56:43	3:53:26
5:33	27:45	55:30	1:57:04	3:54:08
5:34	27:50	55:40	1:57:25	3:54:50
5:35	27:55	55:50	1:57:46	3:55:32
5:36	28:00	56:00	1:58:07	3:56:14
5:37	28:05	56:10	1:58:28	3:56:57
5:38	28:10	56:20	1:58:49	3:57:39
5:39	28:15	56:30	1:59:11	3:58:21

MM:SS/MI	5K	10K	HALF-MARATHON	MARATHON
5:40	28:20	56:40	1:59:32	3:59:03
5:41	28:25	56:50	1:59:53	3:59:45
5:42	28:30	57:00	2:00:14	4:00:28
5:43	28:35	57:10	2:00:35	4:01:10
5:44	28:40	57:20	2:00:56	4:01:52
5:45	28:45	57:30	2:01:17	4:02:34
5:46	28:50	57:40	2:01:38	4:03:16
5:47	28:55	57:50	2:01:59	4:03:59
5:48	29:00	58:00	2:02:20	4:04:41
5:49	29:05	58:10	2:02:41	4:05:23
5:50	29:10	58:20	2:03:03	4:06:05
5:51	29:15	58:30	2:03:24	4:06:47
5:52	29:20	58:40	2:03:45	4:07:29
5:53	29:25	58:50	2:04:06	4:08:12
5:54	29:30	59:00	2:04:27	4:08:54
5:55	29:35	59:10	2:04:48	4:09:36
5:56	29:40	59:20	2:05:09	4:10:18
5:57	29:45	59:30	2:05:30	4:11:00
5:58	29:50	59:40	2:05:51	4:11:43
5:59	29:55	59:50	2:06:12	4:12:25
6:00	30:00	1:00:00	2:06:33	4:13:07
6:01	30:05	1:00:10	2:06:55	4:13:49
6:02	30:10	1:00:20	2:07:16	4:14:31
6:03	30:15	1:00:30	2:07:37	4:15:14
6:04	30:20	1:00:40	2:07:58	4:15:56
6:05	30:25	1:00:50	2:08:19	4:16:38

MM:SS/MI	5K	10K	HALF-MARATHON	MARATHON
6:06	30:30	1:01:00	2:08:40	4:17:20
6:07	30:35	1:01:10	2:09:01	4:18:02
6:08	30:40	1:01:20	2:09:22	4:18:44
6:09	30:45	1:01:30	2:09:43	4:19:27
6:10	30:50	1:01:40	2:10:04	4:20:09
6:11	30:55	1:01:50	2:10:26	4:20:51
6:12	31:00	1:02:00	2:10:47	4:21:33
6:13	31:05	1:02:10	2:11:08	4:22:15
6:14	31:10	1:02:20	2:11:29	4:22:58
6:15	31:15	1:02:30	2:11:50	4:23:40
6:16	31:20	1:02:40	2:12:11	4:24:22
6:17	31:25	1:02:50	2:12:32	4:25:04
6:18	31:30	1:03:00	2:12:53	4:25:46
6:19	31:35	1:03:10	2:13:14	4:26:28
6:20	31:40	1:03:20	2:13:35	4:27:11
6:21	31:45	1:03:30	2:13:56	4:27:53
6:22	31:50	1:03:40	2:14:18	4:28:35
6:23	31:55	1:03:50	2:14:39	4:29:17
6:24	32:00	1:04:00	2:15:00	4:29:59
6:25	32:05	1:04:10	2:15:21	4:30:42
6:26	32:10	1:04:20	2:15:42	4:31:24
6:27	32:15	1:04:30	2:16:03	4:32:06
6:28	32:20	1:04:40	2:16:24	4:32:48
6:29	32:25	1:04:50	2:16:45	4:33:30
6:30	32:30	1:05:00	2:17:06	4:34:13
6:31	32:35	1:05:10	2:17:27	4:34:55

MM:SS/MI	5K	10K	HALF-MARATHON	MARATHON
6:32	32:40	1:05:20	2:17:48	4:35:37
6:33	32:45	1:05:30	2:18:10	4:36:19
6:34	32:50	1:05:40	2:18:31	4:37:01
6:35	32:55	1:05:50	2:18:52	4:37:43
6:36	33:00	1:06:00	2:19:13	4:38:26
6:37	33:05	1:06:10	2:19:34	4:39:08
6:38	33:10	1:06:20	2:19:55	4:39:50
6:39	33:15	1:06:30	2:20:16	4:40:32
6:40	33:20	1:06:40	2:20:37	4:41:14
6:41	33:25	1:06:50	2:20:58	4:41:57
6:42	33:30	1:07:00	2:21:19	4:42:39
6:43	33:35	1:07:10	2:21:40	4:43:21
6:44	33:40	1:07:20	2:22:02	4:44:03
6:45	33:45	1:07:30	2:22:23	4:44:45
6:46	33:50	1:07:40	2:22:44	4:45:28
6:47	33:55	1:07:50	2:23:05	4:46:10
6:48	34:00	1:08:00	2:23:26	4:46:52
6:49	34:05	1:08:10	2:23:47	4:47:34
6:50	34:10	1:08:20	2:24:08	4:48:16
6:51	34:15	1:08:30	2:24:29	4:48:58
6:52	34:20	1:08:40	2:24:50	4:49:41
6:53	34:25	1:08:50	2:25:11	4:50:23
6:54	34:30	1:09:00	2:25:33	4:51:05
6:55	34:35	1:09:10	2:25:54	4:51:47
6:56	34:40	1:09:20	2:26:15	4:52:29
6:57	34:45	1:09:30	2:26:36	4:53:12

MM:SS/MI	5K	10K	HALF-MARATHON	MARATHON
6:58	34:50	1:09:40	2:26:57	4:53:54
6:59	34:55	1:09:50	2:27:18	4:54:36
7:00	35:00	1:10:00	2:27:39	4:55:18
7:01	35:05	1:10:10	2:28:00	4:56:00
7:02	35:10	1:10:20	2:28:21	4:56:42
7:03	35:15	1:10:30	2:28:42	4:57:25
7:04	35:20	1:10:40	2:29:03	4:58:07
7:05	35:25	1:10:50	2:29:25	4:58:49
7:06	35:30	1:11:00	2:29:46	4:59:31
7:07	35:35	1:11:10	2:30:07	5:00:13
7:08	35:40	1:11:20	2:30:28	5:00:56
7:09	35:45	1:11:30	2:30:49	5:01:38
7:10	35:50	1:11:40	2:31:10	5:02:20
7:11	35:55	1:11:50	2:31:31	5:03:02
7:12	36:00	1:12:00	2:31:52	5:03:44
7:13	36:05	1:12:10	2:32:13	5:04:27
7:14	36:10	1:12:20	2:32:34	5:05:09
7:15	36:15	1:12:30	2:32:55	5:05:51
7:16	36:20	1:12:40	2:33:17	5:06:33
7:17	36:25	1:12:50	2:33:38	5:07:15
7:18	36:30	1:13:00	2:33:59	5:07:57
7:19	36:35	1:13:10	2:34:20	5:08:40
7:20	36:40	1:13:20	2:34:41	5:09:22
7:21	36:45	1:13:30	2:35:02	5:10:04
7:22	36:50	1:13:40	2:35:23	5:10:46
7:23	36:55	1:13:50	2:35:44	5:11:28

MM:SS/MI	5K	10K	HALF-MARATHON	MARATHON
7:24	37:00	1:14:00	2:36:05	5:12:11
7:25	37:05	1:14:10	2:36:26	5:12:53
7:26	37:10	1:14:20	2:36:47	5:13:35
7:27	37:15	1:14:30	2:37:09	5:14:17
7:28	37:20	1:14:40	2:37:30	5:14:59
7:29	37:25	1:14:50	2:37:51	5:15:42
7:30	37:30	1:15:00	2:38:12	5:16:24
7:31	37:35	1:15:10	2:38:33	5:17:06
7:32	37:40	1:15:20	2:38:54	5:17:48
7:33	37:45	1:15:30	2:39:15	5:18:30
7:34	37:50	1:15:40	2:39:36	5:19:12
7:35	37:55	1:15:50	2:39:57	5:19:55
7:36	38:00	1:16:00	2:40:18	5:20:37
7:37	38:05	1:16:10	2:40:40	5:21:19
7:38	38:10	1:16:20	2:41:01	5:22:01
7:39	38:15	1:16:30	2:41:22	5:22:43
7:40	38:20	1:16:40	2:41:43	5:23:26
7:41	38:25	1:16:50	2:42:04	5:24:08
7:42	38:30	1:17:00	2:42:25	5:24:50
7:43	38:35	1:17:10	2:42:46	5:25:32
7:44	38:40	1:17:20	2:43:07	5:26:14
7:45	38:45	1:17:30	2:43:28	5:26:56
7:46	38:50	1:17:40	2:43:49	5:27:39
7:47	38:55	1:17:50	2:44:10	5:28:21
7:48	39:00	1:18:00	2:44:32	5:29:03
7:49	39:05	1:18:10	2:44:53	5:29:45

MM:SS/MI	5K	10K	HALF-MARATHON	MARATHON
7:50	39:10	1:18:20	2:45:14	5:30:27
7:51	39:15	1:18:30	2:45:35	5:31:10
7:52	39:20	1:18:40	2:45:56	5:31:52
7:53	39:25	1:18:50	2:46:17	5:32:34
7:54	39:30	1:19:00	2:46:38	5:33:16
7:55	39:35	1:19:10	2:46:59	5:33:58
7:56	39:40	1:19:20	2:47:20	5:34:41
7:57	39:45	1:19:30	2:47:41	5:35:23
7:58	39:50	1:19:40	2:48:02	5:36:05
7:59	39:55	1:19:50	2:48:24	5:36:47
8:00	40:00	1:20:00	2:48:45	5:37:29
8:01	40:05	1:20:10	2:49:06	5:38:11
8:02	40:10	1:20:20	2:49:27	5:38:54
8:03	40:15	1:20:30	2:49:48	5:39:36

ACKNOWLEDGMENTS

For more than 35 years, I have had the pleasure and benefit of collaborating with Scott Murr. Our unending conversations have enriched my understanding of human performance. Scott and I have not only shared thousands of runs, together, we have made many presentations, conducted clinics, published research, and coauthored four books. We have been fortunate to share many gratifying experiences.

In 2003, Scott and I, along with Ray Moss, established the Furman Institute of Running & Scientific Training, which led to the publication of *Run Less Run Faster* in 2007. A revision of the book was published in 2012. Dr. Moss, now retired, was a coauthor of the earlier editions. We appreciate the support and encouragement given to us by Rodale for those earlier editions.

Scott and I have relied on our longtime running partner, editor, and collaborator on all of our projects—my brother, Don. I would not have considered a revision of the book without his willingness to partner again in its development. As in the first two editions, his editing and preparation of tables were an immense contribution.

Amby Burfoot has not only been invaluable to FIRST for his guidance and wisdom, he has been a personal inspiration. Amby is among the world's most knowledgeable people about running. It's a treat to visit with him and learn about the many facets of running. As any serious runner knows, he is incredibly talented, but you would absolutely never know that from talking with him. He is an intellectual who communicates well with the common man. His contributions to the running world are surpassed by no one. We are truly grateful for having the opportunity to be his friend.

Much of what we have learned for this revision has come from our FIRST Running Retreats. Those retreats have been enhanced by several FIRST Retreat faculty members. Mickey McCauley, Furman University assistant track coach, has been with FIRST since its inception.

As a senior at Furman University, Jill Lucas did an independent study project under my supervision that led to the creation of the FIRST Running Retreat. During her independent study, I recognized both her organizational skills and enthusiasm for running. After graduating from Furman, Jill earned graduate degrees in exercise physiology. Dr. Jill Lucas is now an exercise science professor at the University of Lynchburg. She has been a major contributor to our Running Retreats since their inception.

Dr. Phil Gregory, Furman Sports Medicine physical therapist, provided the descriptions of injuries and treatments in Chapter 11. He lectures and performs gait analyses at our Running Retreats. We continue to learn about injury prevention and treatment from his expertise.

Robert Gary, two-time Olympian in the steeplechase, and head coach of Furman's men's and women's cross-country and track teams, graciously provided the foreword for this book. Recently, Robert served as the head coach of the USA men's track and field team at the 2019 World Championships in Doha.

In 2006, I received a cold call from Barrett Neville, at the time a New York City book agent, asking if I had considered writing a book. He had read an article in the *Wall Street Journal* about our FIRST Training Programs. Barrett encouraged and guided us through the process of preparing a book proposal and shopping it to publishers. We have had a long, positive relationship with him. We appreciate how he made what most authors consider a perplexing process an easy and smooth one for us.

After Penguin Random House (PRH) purchased Rodale Books in 2018, we did not know what that would mean for *Run Less Run Faster (RLRF)*. We were pleased when, soon after the sale, we heard from PRH, expressing support for the continued promotion of the 2012 edition and an interest in a third edition. We greatly appreciate all the efforts of Danielle Curtis in clarifying the formal rights to *RLRF* between Rodale and PRH. We are grateful for her persistent pursuit of a third edition of *RLRF*. Danielle contributed valuable recommendations and keen editing. We thank her and PRH for this opportunity.

We rely on our dependable and ever-pleasant administrative assistant, Lonita Stegall, for communications with FIRST clients and the preparation of materials for our presentations and clinics.

We have been fortunate to interact with runners from all six inhabited continents. It's been a joy to learn about their challenges and successes. Those interactions have shaped our ideas and our programs. We continue to strive to develop programs and offer services to promote running as a healthy, safe, and fun activity.

Bill Pierce

3. Realistic Goals

1. Gina Kolata, "Staying a Step Ahead of Aging," *New York Times* (January 31, 2008), https://www.nytimes.com/2008/01/31/health/nutrition/31BEST.html

2. W. M. Bortz IV & W. M. Bortz II, "How Fast Do We Age? Exercise Performance over Time as Biomarker," *Journal of Gerontology. Series A, Biological Sciences and Medical Sciences* 51, no. 5 (1996), M223–M225.

3. Ibid.

4. S. Murr & B. Pierce, "How Aging Impacts Runners' Goals of Lifelong Running," *Physical Activity and Health* 3, no. 1 (2019), 71–81. doi: http://doi.org/10.5334/paah.42.

10. Altitude Training and Racing

1. Benjamin D. Levine and James Stray-Gundersen, " 'Living High–Training Low': Effect of Moderate-Altitude Acclimatization with Low-Altitude Training on Performance," *Journal of Applied Physiology* (July 1997). https://doi.org/10.1152/jappl.1997.83.1.102.

2. J. Ness, "Is Live High/Train Low the Ultimate Endurance Training Model?" *NSCA Coach*, 2, Issue 1 (January 2013). https://www.nsca.com/education/articles/nsca-coach/is-live-hightrain-low-the-ultimate-endurance-training-model/.

3. A. Baker & W. G. Hopkins, "Altitude Training for Sea-Level Competition," *Sportscience Training & Technology* (1998). Internet Society for Sport Science. http://sportsci.org/traintech/altitude/wgh.html.

4. E. Beresini, "Do Altitude Tents Work?" *Outside* (May 24, 2013). https://www.outsideonline.com/1784286/do-altitude-tents-work.

13. Body Composition

1. Scott Murr & Bill Pierce, "How Aging Impacts Runners' Goals of Lifelong Running," *Physical Activity and Health* (2019): 3(1), 71–81. https://paahjournal.com/articles/10.5334/paah.42/.

2. Ibid.

3. Ibid.

14. Strength Training for Runners

1. "Preserve Your Muscle Mass," *Harvard Health Publishing*, February 2016. https://www.health.harvard.edu/staying-healthy/preserve-your-muscle-mass.

2. F. Brunner, A. Schmid, A. Sheikhzadeh, M. Nordin, J. Yoon, and V. Frankel, "Effects of Aging on Type II Muscle Fibers: A Systematic Review of the Literature," *Journal of Aging and Physical Activity* 15, no. 3 (July 2007): 336–48.

Protein, 186
Push-ups (standard or modified), 214